The Theory and Practice of Relational Coaching

D1548275

The 'relational turn' is a movement affecting a range of disciplines including neuroscience, psychoanalysis, psychotherapy, organisational consulting and, more recently, coaching. Its primary focus is on the centrality of human relating in determining how individuals develop, make meaning and function individually and collectively.

In *The Theory and Practice of Relational Coaching: Complexity, Paradox and Integration*, Simon Cavicchia and Maria Gilbert expand existing coaching theory and practice to focus on the implications of the relational turn for how coaches and clients think about the nature of identity, the self, change, learning, and individual and organisational development. Drawing on perspectives as varied as relational neuroscience, the relational foundations of personality development, psychoanalysis, psychotherapy, shame, vulnerability, complexity and systems ideas, the authors shed light on many of the paradoxes and challenges facing coaches and their clients in today's fast-paced, volatile and uncertain organisational environments. These include holding tensions such as the uniqueness of individual needs with the requirements of organisational contexts, managing multiple stakeholder expectations and networks and balancing linear approaches to change with adjusting to emerging and unpredictable events.

Given the ever-increasing volatility, complexity and uncertainty that coaches and their clients face, *The Theory and Practice of Relational Coaching* guides the reader through a series of illuminating perspectives, examples and practical suggestions. These will enable coaches to integrate a more relational orientation in their work and extend their range and that of their clients for responding creatively to the challenges of modern organisational life. The book will appeal to coaches and coaching psychologists in practice and training, as well as counsellors and psychotherapists retraining as coaches.

Simon Cavicchia is an executive coach, a UKCP registered Gestalt psychotherapist, consultant and supervisor. He was Joint Programme Leader of the MSc in Coaching Psychology at the Metanoia Institute in London for eight years. He divides his time between executive coaching, consulting and teaching on postgraduate programmes in coaching and organisational development. He is currently on the faculty of the Ashridge Masters in Executive Coaching.

Maria Gilbert is a Chartered Clinical Psychologist, a UKCP registered Integrative psychotherapist, BACP accredited supervisor and coach. For many years, she was the Joint Head of the Integrative Department, the Supervision Training and the MSc in Coaching Psychology at the Metanoia Institute in London, and a Visiting Professor at Middlesex University.

The Theory and Practice of Relational Coaching

Complexity, Paradox and Integration

Simon Cavicchia and
Maria Gilbert

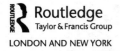

Routledge
Taylor & Francis Group

LONDON AND NEW YORK

First published 2019
by Routledge
2 Park Square, Milton Park, Abingdon, Oxon OX14 4RN

and by Routledge
711 Third Avenue, New York, NY 10017

Routledge is an imprint of the Taylor & Francis Group, an informa business

British Library Cataloguing-in-Publication Data
A catalogue record for this book is available from the British Library

Library of Congress Cataloging-in-Publication Data
Names: Cavicchia, Simon, author. | Gilbert, Maria, author.
Title: The theory and practice of relational coaching : complexity,
paradox and integration / Simon Cavicchia and Maria Gilbert.
Description: New York : Routledge, 2018. | Includes bibliographical
references and index.
Identifiers: LCCN 2018007732 (print) | LCCN 2018013197 (ebook) |
ISBN 9780429469510 (Master e-book) | ISBN 9780415643245 (hardback :
alk. paper) | ISBN 9780415643252 (pbk. : alk. paper) | ISBN 9780429469510 (ebk)
Subjects: LCSH: Counseling. | Interpersonal relations—Psychological aspects.
Classification: LCC BF636.6 (ebook) | LCC BF636.6 .C38 2018 (print) |
DDC 158.3—dc23
LC record available at https://lccn.loc.gov/2018007732

ISBN: 978-0-415-64324-5 (hbk)
ISBN: 978-0-415-64325-2 (pbk)
ISBN: 978-0-429-46951-0 (ebk)

Typeset in Times New Roman
by Florence Production Ltd, Stoodleigh, Devon, UK

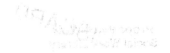

Contents

Acknowledgements

There are many individuals who have been instrumental in the writing of this book and to whom we wish to express particular thanks. Our clients who have shared of themselves and their challenges, and from whom we continue to learn so much. Our students and coaching supervisees over the years with whom many of the ideas we explore have been tested and refined in light of their honest feedback as practitioners. Molly Rawle at the *International Gestalt Journal* for permission to use a paper Simon originally published in 2009 as the basis for Chapter 11. Alper Eroglu, Robin Hindle Fisher, Jason Harrison, Anne-Marie Lawlor, Sandy Nelson and Charlotte Sills for reading early drafts of chapters and providing suggestions and insights from both client and practitioner perspectives. Ruth Windle for supervision, insight and offering permission, acceptance and space to explore. The editorial team at Routledge for the ease and care with which you have managed the relationship with us.

Finally, from Simon, a heartfelt thanks to my husband Fabrice who is my greatest relationship teacher.

A note on the text

A word about case examples

All the examples in this book are drawn from real events, situations and dynamics that have arisen in the context of coaching with a relational and integrative orientation. Examples have been created by combining different elements which frequently arise in coaching situations but have been written in a way that does not identify any specific individual or organisation.

A word about language

The pronouns he and she have been used equally throughout the book. We have used coachee and client interchangeably to mean the individual recipient of the coaching.

Section 1

The relational turn and coaching

Chapter I

Setting the scene for an integrative relational approach to coaching in challenging times

Uncertainty, paradox and complexity

We live in complex times. The technological advances of the internet have resulted in unprecedented levels of human connection across time and distance. At the same time, technology, with its corresponding speed and volume of data traffic, is also giving rise to human disconnection. It can become a substitute for more direct human contact and the more subtle qualities of human relating, where, instead of talking and thinking together, colleagues sitting opposite one another resort to transacting primarily via email.

For some time seismic shifts have been occurring in global institutions and belief systems. Whatever different individuals may feel and think to this day, the last 150 years have seen a series of significant developments in relation to the social construction of ethnicity, power, sex and sexuality. It is only a hundred years ago that women did not have equal voting rights to men in the United Kingdom. It is relatively recently that apartheid has given way to the beginnings of a more inclusive democracy in South Africa, and more recently still that America saw its first black president in Barack Obama. While questions have been asked in some quarters for some time about the often idealistic, reductionist and taken for granted assumptions underpinning capitalism as an ideology (Eisenstein, 2011), the global financial crisis of recent years has resulted in dialogue about both the benefits and shadows of market forces to be aired on an unprecedented scale in the global arena. This dialogue continues at the time of writing this book (Heffernan, 2014; Picketty, 2014). There is not the scope here to discuss the many potential ramifications of these shifts for our species and planet. We believe these will be revealed and worked out over time, and are an inevitable part of the evolution of human thought and the emerging meanings, priorities and behaviours this gives rise to. We want, however, to point to the ways in which constructs and meanings, which may have hitherto provided a sense (albeit illusory) of security and predictability, also inevitably undergo re-working in light of new experiences, perspectives and discourse. This is also true of coaching itself as a profession and practice.

As the world reveals itself to be characterised by ever increasing uncertainty, individuals and groups are drawing on the vast potential for humans, as fundamentally social beings, to make meaning together and strategise for collective survival and well-being, as in the case of the sustainability movement. For some, uncertainty provides freedom from the constraining elements of past beliefs and constructs that are revealing themselves to be, at best, unreliable in conferring predictability and stability, and at worst, overly limiting or even harmful. Uncertainty, and the disequilibrium this gives rise to, can support a re-evaluation of working assumptions, an antidote to short termism (Nowotny, 2016) and the creation of new meanings and practices that might lean more towards community, inclusion and the exploration of differences in service of understanding, co-operation and the generation of new knowledge. For others, uncertainty gives rise to deep anxieties in the face of the questioning of sincere and long held beliefs. This can result in a rigidifying of existing positions and a retreat into individual isolation, or tightly policed homogenised groups, where membership is predicated on unquestioning compliance with group think, community and organisational norms.

A little closer to the context of coaching, organisation theory has evolved from the mechanistic assumptions of the early 1900s (Gilbreth, 1911; Taylor, 1911). Here organisations were conceptualised as machines and human capital as units to be manipulated in the service of organisational goals. For many years these models persisted and appeared fit for purpose due to the influence of, and compliance with, socially constructed and enforced assumptions about productivity, power and hierarchy. While these assumptions are still very influential, since the turn of the last century, organisations have also begun to be seen as complex fields of human interaction and social processes (Eoyang, 2013; Oshry, 2007; Shaw, 2002; Stacey, 2001). From this perspective, meaning and resulting behaviour is being constantly constructed through the participation and conversations of organisation members. It is in these conversations also that different meanings about the purpose and nature of work are emerging. Younger generations of employees hold different assumptions about the place of work in their lives and the psychological contract they look for with their employers (Hobart and Sendek, 2014). A number of organisations are also asking questions about the nature of the bottom line and how to measure an organisation's value not simply in terms of profit and shareholder dividends. For some, contribution to the wider societies in which they operate, the well-being of employees and environmental sustainability are increasingly coming to be seen as values based currency (Willard, 2012; Laszlo and Zhexembayeva, 2011). These latter concerns are also consistent with the emergence of a more complex and inclusive consciousness as has been described by researchers of adult development such as Wilber (2000), Torbert (2004), Graves (2005) and Cook-Greuter (2004). Laloux (2014) has examined the ways in which this emerging consciousness, characterised by lifelong learning, less individual ego motivated behaviour, greater appreciation of complexity and interconnectedness, is manifesting in individuals and the organisations they create. He points to the ways in which these characteristics are vital in being able to respond creatively to more complex problems that cannot be resolved, as Einstein is purported to have stated, at the same level of consciousness that created them.

The VUCA world

In the 1990s the acronym VUCA began to appear first in military and later organisational writing to describe environments where leaders and those who participate in organisational life are facing unprecedented volatility, uncertainty, complexity and ambiguity (Stiehm and Townsend, 2002). Past models and processes are no longer adequate to contain and navigate these challenges, and leaders are often faced with the dilemma of not knowing how best to proceed, having only ever partial information, but needing, nonetheless, to act. Adjusting to and navigating these challenges calls on individuals to know themselves better, manage their own feelings of anxiety, bear uncertainty, take up fluid roles, experience shifts in personal identity, and continue to be able to think, reflect, make sense and act under pressure (Hirschhorn, 1998; Kegan, 1994). Reliance on rigid processes, protocols and control mechanisms is no longer sufficient in many organisational contexts given the challenges they face, and in some, these mechanisms actually cause and perpetuate structural difficulties and less than productive behaviours (Laloux, 2014; Schwartz, 1990).

There is now a greater need for individuals to come together, relate differently and effectively in order to create new ways of thinking, being, working and organising. This requires the harnessing of difference, fostering greater aware ness of, and critical reflection on, the assumptions that underpin current thinking and action. It calls for paying close attention to the quality of connection and conversation between individuals, groups and entire organisations in order to develop the effectiveness, agility and responsiveness today's business, societal and global challenges call for (Lines and Scholes–Rhodes, 2013).

The unfolding of coaching – Identity crisis or integrative opportunity?

Coaching too is undergoing rapid theoretical expansion which is inevitably informing how coaching is embodied and delivered by practitioners. From the GROW model of the early 1990s and similar protocol and technique based approaches, the field of coaching now includes, among many perspectives, increased openness to psychological understanding (Palmer and Whybrow, 2011), systems thinking (O'Neill, 2007; Whittington, 2012), complexity perspectives (Cavanagh, 2006), somatic (Strozzi-Heckler, 2014), ontological (Olalla, 2010; Sieler, 2010), constructivist-developmental (Bachkirova, 2010) and transpersonal perspectives (Rowan, 2010). The focus for many years on hard individual behavioural goals is being deconstructed and revealing itself to be more subtle, complex and both potentially useful in bringing focus, while also problematic in narrowing perspectives on a complex set of presenting issues and contexts (Boyatzis and Howard, 2013; Cavanagh, 2013; De Haan, 2014; Grant, 2013).

In the time we have been working as coaches there have been a number of shifts in the construction and conceptualisation of the profession. From early attempts to define coaching as very distinct and different from other talking developmental relationships, and a suspicion of anything psychological, to an appreciation and increased acknowledgement of the debt early coaching approaches owe not just to adult learning theory and pragmatism (Cox, 2013), but also the science and art of psychology, counselling and psychotherapy (Cox, Bachkirova and Clutterbuck, 2011; Palmer and Whybrow, 2007). Increasingly clients and sponsors are being exposed to the potential benefits of psychological mindedness in the context of coaching, and some accrediting bodies such as the Association of Professional Executive Coaching and Supervision (APECS) in the United Kingdom consider a degree of psychological understanding to be a necessary component in executive coaching. Popovic and Jinks (2013) have coined the expression 'personal consultancy' and set out the beginnings of a model which attempts to consciously integrate the coaching and counselling paradigms and professions. While many of the challenges and paradoxes inherent in an integrative project of this kind are still to be worked out, and may never be fully resolved, it is encouraging to us that so many new possibilities, challenges and questions are being asked.

Current and existing definitions of coaching tend to be very general and high level. Within them there is a vast range of freedom and scope for coaches 'in practice' to develop a unique approach to coaching based on their own personalities, training, histories and life experience, all interacting with these corresponding aspects and unique requirements in their different clients and their contexts.

An integrative-relational orientation is one particular perspective which we believe has much to offer and is in keeping with post modernity, the challenges of our times and the VUCA world. We certainly do not wish to suggest that this is the only way, nor do we believe to have resolved all of the tensions and challenges inherent in an approach of this kind. Yet we do believe in the potential of integration and a relational turn for bringing much to coaching and the world of human development through the medium of human interaction.

As coaching as a profession matures, and the focus moves from defining to refining, there seems to be a movement towards locating coaching in a wider body of theory, research and systems of thought than were first acknowledged as influential (Western, 2017, 2012). Professionalism can no longer be assumed simply on the basis of the acquisition and practicing of skills, which has been the primary vehicle for coach training, development and accreditation in some quarters. Instead it needs also to be predicated on broader experience, self-awareness and the personal maturity and reflexivity required to navigate the complexities of client issues and their contexts. Skills and techniques are important, but if we limit the notion of professionalism primarily to the demonstrable acquisition of skills, rigid adherence to the preferred protocols of specific accrediting bodies, and hours clocked up in the driving seat, we risk missing the subtlety, nuances and creativity that can be made use of when we consciously acknowledge and widen the theoretical and practice foundation upon which professionalism in action is based.

The construction of coaching, coach and coachee

The early differentiation between coaching and psychological therapies is understandable in terms of coaching and coach training being oriented towards working with clients seeking to develop personally and professionally, but where there are no apparent symptoms of mental illness. This demarcation also supported the establishment of coaching as a distinct profession with the attendant risk that vested interests, commercial opportunities, schoolism, professionalism and professionalisation become ends in themselves, codifying, rigidifying and ultimately losing the vibrancy and transformative potential of ongoing theoretical and practice evolution.

The emergence of coaching early on in the context of sport and organisational life has meant that it implicitly comes to reflect many of the central concerns of these fields of endeavour such as winning, being the best, translating coaching practices into quick results, clear and value-adding material terms. While these objectives undoubtedly have their place, and can be suited to certain types of coaching such as skills acquisition, performance or development, over-privileging these linear and deterministic biases can lead to a narrowing of what can be considered appropriate or workable in a coaching conversation. The metaphor of the individual leader as a corporate athlete may have much to offer in terms of developing resilience, focus, drive and commitment. However, it can also discount the need for leaders to be orienting to the wider complex social processes, psychological and systemic factors that have a direct bearing on individual and collective capacity, organisational functioning and success. Coaches and coachees, under great social and cultural pressure to be able to instantly apply learning and demonstrate their respective worth, can find it difficult to allow the time and space necessary for new meanings and strategies to emerge in complex environments.

Fortunately coaching boundaries are expanding to include greater appreciation of the need for meaning making, well-being, complexity and systemic perspectives. These are particularly suited to executive coaching where coachees are often faced with existential questions, the need for transformational learning and systems understanding if they are to be successful (Hawkins and Smith, 2010). While a relational orientation to coaching can inform all approaches to coaching, it is here that we believe it has a particular contribution to make.

A consequence of earlier constructions of coaching is also the way in which coachees have been constructed. In some texts, the 'ideal' client is seen to be highly motivated to learn, uncomplicatedly aligned with corporate agendas, values and culture, driven to achieve and succeed in particular ways defined by dominant corporate and societal ideologies of the time and place. It is often assumed that he has little or no underlying anxieties or vulnerabilities and can quickly make use of 'established' coaching methods to achieve desired and 'extraordinary' results, thereby fulfilling a contemporary ideal of success, while also reinforcing images of coach competence and the potency of the approach.

Over the years, these constructs have begun to reveal themselves *in practice* to be less clear (Spinelli, 2008). Western (2017, 2012) describes how psychotherapy has often been associated with a 'wounded self' and working to heal from the past, while coaching has been more concerned with the 'celebrated self' and working to develop human potential in individuals with little or no underlying causes of distress or vulnerability. These aspects of human experience have often been polarised in coaching discourse. In some respects this distinction has had its uses such as making for apparently simple discrimination between professions and ensuring that those lacking the training to work at psychological depth are not working beyond the limits of their capability.

Once we shift our viewing angle from abstract theoretical discussion to looking closely at what happens in the moment by moment relational interactions of coach and coachee, many of the distinctions which might appear to hold at the level of theory, professional orthodoxies and schoolism, reveal themselves to be problematic in practice situations. Complexity and human subjectivity mean that clients do encounter uncertainty and vulnerability in the face of complex challenges. These in turn can evoke resistance and patterns of reactivity rooted in early developmental experiences and upbringing. Over-privileging the celebrated self can result in coaches missing opportunities to work with this dimension and can also lead to coaching being used as a sophisticated form of narcissitic supply, shoring up grandiose self images as a defence against vulnerability. Similarly, over-privileging the wounded self, as can be the case in psychotherapy, risks keeping clients focused on deficit and not on their potential. In practice what is often revealed is that vulnerability and potential co-exist in human beings, and often sources of vulnerability and anxiety need to be addressed in order to unlock potential where it is being held back.

Psychotherapists with experience of organisational consulting and coaching have long known that theories and principles of psychotherapy are not only useful for the mentally ill, although they may inform thinking and be deployed differently in organisational contexts. Coaches with the appropriate training and disposition have also worked successfully at greater psychological depth than simply effecting behavioural change and improvements in performance through encouraging clients to generate new options for themselves. In fact, many changes in behaviour, if they are to be meaningful and sustainable, often require working at greater depth (Popovic and Jinks, 2013; Western, 2017, 2012). As coaching theory expands, along with the contexts in which it is being used, theoretical discussion is becoming more subtle and sophisticated. Greater critical reflection is being brought to bear on the nature of the profession, its theoretical, ethical and practice base.

In his study of coaching and mentoring Western (2012) applies four critical frames to his exploration of the coaching profession, each of which illuminates practice from a particular perspective:

Depth analysis

Drawing on psychoanalysis and discourse analysis this orientation works on the premise that much of what happens in human relations and organisational system dynamics happens below the surface in individual and collective unconscious processes.

Emancipation

This is a concern with improving the life of the coachee and acknowledging and exploring tensions and conflicts that might arise between this and the drive in organisations for efficiency, productivity and goals. These 'ends' are often seen to justify 'means' which, if not balanced with regard for the feelings, motivations and well-being of individuals, can result in individual alienation and the dehumanising of the workplace.

Looking awry

This is an orientation which seeks to 'disrupt the normative, to look differently, and discover something new' (Western, 2012, p. 39). It seeks to make room for the coachee's desire, suspend the rational for a while, allow for subjectivity and for new and apparently random associations to be made to support the generation of new knowledge and action strategies.

Network analysis

This seeks to locate coaching in the wider social-political environment. It supports mapping where and how the coachee stands in his or her network, in relation power and powerlessness and the different relationships, forces and patterns that might need to be engaged with and influenced for change to occur.

We believe these are exciting and important perspectives to be bringing to coaching and, as will be seen later, are compatible with an integrative and relational orientation. They are also relatively new developments, which represent an expansion beyond the dominant perspectives and assumptions that have underpinned much coaching theory, practice and training to date.

Modernism, positivism and individualism

The modernist era spanning the late nineteenth to early twentieth centuries is characterised by assumptions based on Newtonian physics, logic, rationality and cause and effect thinking. This era spawned a number of paradigms (a set of assumptions and practices that define a scientific discipline at a given time) such as positivism.

Positivism

Positivism is a school of scientific thought based upon the proposition that information derived from the logical and mathematical treatment of reports of sensory experience is the exclusive source of all authoritative knowledge. Data derived in this way and verified is called empirical evidence of a phenomenon. Other forms of knowing such as the introspective, subjective and intuitive are discounted in this system. Society and human beings are seen to operate, like the physical world, on the basis of general laws.

Individualism

Another characteristic of the modernist era (but with deeper historical roots) is the tendency towards individualism, which chimes with the positivist ideas of individual components interacting according to generalised laws. The main assumption, going back to Plato (Lee and Wheeler, 1997) at the heart of the individualist paradigm is that of separateness. Relationship viewed from within this paradigm is purely instrumental to the expression and gratification of individual needs and drives. Thus the nature of the social world is constructed as subject-object. Here the individual is subject and others are objects to be acted upon, manipulated even, in order for individuals to achieve their goals and desires. This corresponds to the theologian Martin Buber's (1987) description of I-It relating. The subject-object construct also lies at the heart of an expert model of helping (Haslebo and Haslebo, 2012).

It is important not to forget how pervasive, and often unacknowledged, positivist and individualist assumptions are in contemporary thought and the role they have played in shaping coaching theory and practice. It is this pervasiveness that gives rise in coaches and organisation clients alike to a host of assumptions about command and control, communication as a linear form of transmission, where others are expected to immediately understand and heed what is being said or requested, and act accordingly. This explains the frequent frustration, confusion and disorientation when individuals fail to do this. It is the individualist orientation that gives rise to an orientation between coach and coachee of 'doer and done to' (Benjamin, 2004).

Much coaching theory is sensitive to the potential for manipulation and coercion, yet it seems to discount the fact that any coach deploying a suite of tools, which cannot but be the products of a multitude of implicit theoretical and practice assumptions, is inevitably configuring the coaching relationship and direction of travel in a host of subtle and not so subtle ways. This gives rise to an emphasis in some coaching methodologies on systematic procedural approaches with less space for adaptability and spontaneity. Here it is not the coach's role to sit at times with uncertainty and make new meaning *with* a client about his or her situation. The coach is less likely to be seen as someone who also stands to be changed and influenced by the client's subjectivity in a relationship, where new knowledge and possibilities for action cannot be known in advance, but emerge as a function of the exploration and dynamics of interaction. Rather the coach is seen to direct and guide inquiry based on a host of assumptions about how change happens and what might be socially and organisationally desirable, or constitute a requirement of the sponsoring organisation.

A more integrative and relational orientation to coaching, equally, cannot but be shaped by a host of working principles about human development, identity and relational dynamics, but seeks to be increasingly aware of the assumptions underpinning relating and action. It encourages developing the reflexivity to explore different assumptions and the different perspectives and interventions they might give rise to, as well as considering the contextual factors that might be shaping the coaching interaction. It is predicated on a subject-subject construction of the coaching relationship where coach and coachee pay close attention to how they co-create each other's conditions for success (Haslebo and Haslebo, 2012).

Yet from the individualist perspective the coach can still be seen as the causative agent that brings about effects in the client. In some contexts the coach may also be expected to make judgements about a coachee's 'compliance' with the direction of travel established at the contracting phase with relevant parties, hold clients to account and ensure stated parameters are adhered to. From within this paradigm rapport may be considered significant in so much as it enables the coach to steer a trusting client through an established process towards a specified set of outcomes. Where a client seems unable to move in the direction implied by the methodology in use, or stated as desired in the contracting phase, they risk being labeled as resistant, uncoachable or non-compliant. There is, in this construction, likely to be less room to explore and surface the multitude of possible meanings behind an apparent 'lack of compliance', how this perception is being constructed, and what this might have to offer in terms of understanding the factors in coach, client and context that might have a bearing on the coachee's capacity to take effective action.

From within the individualist paradigm agency (the capacity to take action and have impact) is seen to be subjective and to reside within the individual (McNamee and Gergen, 1999). Hence the historical focus in coaching on individual goals. There is likely to be less room for exploring the role of context in shaping client goals, in constructing what is permissible to aim for, and whether the goals a coachee states publicly at the start of an engagement are actually what privately might be desired, or actually be required in order for meaningful, contextually relevant, functional and realistic change to occur. Instead goals have tended to be framed primarily as hard, specific, observable, and, at least partially, knowable in advance based on assumptions about what is considered to be desirable and worth aiming for in the client and their context. Assumptions about change will be mainly predicated on identifying gaps and taking logical steps to do what is believed to be required within a particular theoretical frame to get from A to B. Given the privileging of pragmatism in much coaching theory and practice, the system of the coach-coachee relationship has often been seen primarily as a tightly bounded space in which certain subjects are deemed appropriate and relevant and where others are off limits. The relationship is a place to get things done, and less a more open space in which there might be room for free association and 'play' in order to discover hitherto unforeseen and unimagined new connections, meanings and possibilities for action. This latter orientation is particularly suited to coaching in complex environments where clear and obvious solutions may not be possible, and where coachees are faced with having to resolve in meaningful ways a host of tensions, paradoxes and conflicting priorities in themselves and in their contexts.

Western (2017, 2012) traces the history of coaching and the different influences that have shaped and continue to influence theory and practice to this day. He identifies four dominant discourses, which he describes as a 'socialized way of thinking' (Western, 2012, p. 125), which can be seen to operate in the ongoing emergence of the profession. Each of these discourses influences how coaches perceive coaching and their clients – what he calls the coaching 'gaze'; what coaches actually do in practice, coaching activity and how coaches take up their roles – the coaching 'stance'; and what aspect of the self coaches work on with their clients –the 'object' of the work.

The psy expert discourse

Rooted in modernity this draws on much theory derived from psychology and neuroscience such as cognitive behavioural approaches. The coaching gaze here is focused on performance and there will be an emphasis on goals and outcomes. The coach's stance in relation to the client is to be a 'technician of the psyche' (Western, 2012, p. 250) using tools and techniques to work on cognition and behaviour to enable the client to improve performance and achieve their goals. The object of the work is the 'outward self' (p. 250) of the coachee, how they act and perform, engage with others and are perceived, including working to modify perception through modifying behaviour.

The managerial discourse

Another product of modernism with its values of scientific rigour and rationality, the managerial discourse is concerned primarily with efficiency through control. The gaze is towards 'productivity' (Western, 2012, p. 249) and how to enable the coachee to take up their role and influence others to make their organisation more productive. The coach's stance is to be a 'role coach' (p. 250) exploring with the coachee the various roles he/she may be required by the context to take up, how to do this, how they may be perceived by others, how to manage any tensions there may be between roles and how role is implicated in outputs and effectiveness. The object of the work is for the coachee to work on their 'role self' (p. 251).

The soul guide discourse

For Western (2012) this discourse 'transcends the rational and the material – it enables a playfulness to explore deep human experience in the unique space created by the coaching pair' (p. 132). It has its roots in long established contemplative traditions, spiritual practice and the transpersonal, and yet in relation to coaching 'is the most contemporary approach, taking coaching beyond the discourses of modernity (Psy Expert and Managerial)' (p. 132). The soul guide discourse offers an opportunity to expand the territory of coaching beyond modernity's preoccupations with efficiency and productivity, and therapeutic preoccupations with 'problems' of mental health where clients risk becoming construed as helpless 'patients'. As will be seen, this discourse sits well within a relational orientation to coaching which honours the uniqueness of individual experience, subjectivity, human vulnerability and desire. This discourse 'opens a space to explore the essence of the self – the existential self, the meaning of lives, angst, joy, fear and frailty, hopes and desires, freedom, confinement, values and meaning' (p. 135). The coach's gaze is focused on the client's 'experience' (p. 249). There is a focus on the subjective and bodily experience of both coach and coachee in the here and now. The coach will use his or her experience of being with the coachee to relate to the client, understand his or her experience and facilitate learning from what is arising in the present moment. The coach's stance is to be a 'mirror to the soul' (p. 250). This is challenging in that it involves resisting the pull into activity or technique characteristic of the previous two discourses. Instead it privileges abiding more in the present moment, opening to direct experience, intuition, speaking from this place and trusting in the process of being with an other as it unfolds for what it can offer in terms of learning and insight. We shall elaborate further on this process in Section 2. The object of the work is for the coachee to work on their 'inner self' (p. 250), their feelings, any anxiety, vulnerabilities and concerns. It supports clients to discover what they desire and how they can find purpose and meaning. As such it is concerned with existential questions, identity and well-being and also resonates with practices associated with the evolution of consciousness as set out by Wilber (2000) and Laloux (2014).

The network coach discourse

This discourse 'takes coaching beyond individual psychology, soul work or performance and situates the individual in the networks of work and society' (Western, 2012, p. 13). Western sees this as the newest discourse emerging in coaching, which has a vital role 'in shifting coaching from personal and operational interventions towards strategic thinking that also takes an ethical stance' (p. 13). As such this discourse sits comfortably within a relational orientation with its emphasis on the interconnectedness and mutually influencing dynamics of individuals and their contexts, and an openness to intersubjectivity, multiple meanings and complexity. The coach's gaze is directed at this 'connectivity' (p. 249) helping clients to locate themselves in the networks of culture and activity they inhabit. It is concerned with helping clients identify where they might influence, who they might need to connect up and connect with in order for change to occur. It is also the discourse that takes an ethical perspective (unlike the assumed neutrality of the modernist scientific methods underpinning the psy expert and managerial discourses) and is concerned with enabling the coachee to make connections between their values, those of the company, their work and the wider social and environmental context. The coach's stance is to be an 'emergent strategist' (p. 250) not getting bogged down in operational detail but supporting the coachee to access and maintain an open, reflective and generative mindset. The coach supports the coachee to identify patterns that lead to emergent strategies, improve interactions with stakeholders, experiment with new business models and spot new opportunities. This is an inherently relational orientation where the coachee works on their 'networked self' (p. 251), identifying where and how they are located in their network(s). Coach and coachee work to identify patterns, explore how the coachee is shaped by and relates to different contexts, understands and responds to the different connections and influences in their network which could be people as well as technology, ideology and cultural forces.

We shall expand on this from our own perspective and relational orientation in subsequent chapters.

Post modernism and the relational turn

The 'relational turn', as it has come to be known, is a movement affecting a range of disciplines including neuroscience, psychoanalysis and psychotherapy, modern physics, organisational consulting and, more recently, coaching. It is characterised by an increasing interest in the dynamics of human relating and their centrality in determining how individuals develop, make meaning, function and take action in the world (Clarke et al., 2008). De Haan and Sills (2012) have summarised a number of factors that contribute to this evolving trend.

Developments in neuroscience have revealed the way in which early relationships and interactions have a profound impact on the development of a stable and coherent sense of self which then affects the capacity for stability and functioning in adult life (Fonagy, Gergely, Jurist, Target, 2002). Fonagy et al. (2002) go on to show how early relational patterns become a template for later relating, meaning making and behaviour in the world. Early experiences of being attuned to empathically by an 'other', usually a parent or primary caregiver, lay the foundations for the capacity to empathise with others and appreciate multiple subjectivities, differing experiences and perspectives, without feeling threatened or needing to control the minds of others through imposing one single perspective as if this were the only truth.

Organisational thinkers (Stacey, 1992, 2001; Macintosh *et al.*, 2006; Streatfield, 2001; Shaw, 2002; Shaw and Stacey, 2006) conceive of organisations not as structural mechanistic entities, but as complex subjective webs of communicative interaction, where patterns of thought and action emerge, amplify and dissolve.

Meaning itself is seen to be a function of relationship. Quantum physics describes the influence of the perspective of the observer on the outcome of observation – how we look determines what we see (Mindell, 2000). Perspectives from the field of social constructionism point to the co-created and contextual nature of how meaning is made and knowledge generated (Burr, 2003; Gergen, 2009). Research into human relating highlights the potency of intersubjectivity, the reciprocal process of influencing that goes on, moment by moment, in all relationships and conversations (Stolorow and Atwood, 1992).

In depth effectiveness studies in psychotherapy (Horvath and Symonds, 1991; Martin, Garske and Davis, 2000; Norcross, 2011) have identified the central importance of the quality of relationship between practitioner and client in determining the success of helping relationships. The quality of relationship is seen as a more consistent indicator of success than any particular theoretical school or orientation. Wampold (2001) highlights a number of key relational elements considered important for the working alliance between client and therapist including the client's 'affectionate' relationship with the practitioner; the client's motivation and ability to work collaboratively with the therapist; the therapist's empathic responding to, flexibility and involvement with the client. While the foci and contexts of coaching may differ in some respects from psychotherapy, we shall explore these perspectives for what they may also have to offer coaches and coachees.

The relational turn represents a significant shift in paradigm from the positivist and individualist traditions. It makes central a focus on the relationship between people, ideologies, social forces, patterns and ideas. It spans different scientific and ideological territories and systems of thought including the psychological territory of human experience and relating, the sociological territory of human organisation and behaviour and the ecological and wider community connections that shape the unfolding of meaning and well-being of the planet and its inhabitants. A relational orientation can be applied at different levels of system, including the dynamics of the coach-coachee dyad and how these can be utilised in the service of learning and change; the ways coachees and their clients think about, conceptualise and participate in organisations and relationship patterns at work; the wider purpose of the project of coaching itself and its potential role in shaping understanding, learning, development and consciousness.

Social constructionism

The relational turn is essentially a product of the post-modern era where rigid attachment to ideas related to scientific certainty, objective measurement and universal laws is now being met with an increased opening to multiplicity and subjectivity. Here there is greater appreciation of knowledge and knowing that is not necessarily empirically demonstrable yet nonetheless holds great meaning and significance for people, and powerfully guides thinking and behaviour. In post modernity 'we have become sceptical about grand narratives, where there are no universally agreed beliefs . . . where everything is therefore contingent' (Western, 2012, p. 101). The questioning characteristic of post-modernism can offer tremendous opportunities for innovation and creativity while also increasing anxiety and uncertainty. Western (2012) suggests that in this post modern landscape there is a greater need for friendship and relational connection as this enables us to have intimacy while also maintaining the 'nomadic autonomy' demanded in the post-modern world. We see this as another important reason why a relational orientation to coaching has much to offer both in terms of human to human support and creating conditions where coachees can be helped to make their own sense of complexity and plot their own courses through their organisations and lives.

Out of this tradition a particular orientation to knowledge and meaning making has emerged which warrants attention here – the field of social constructionism. This particular way of thinking about knowledge or 'epistemology' holds that nothing can really be objectively known because, as the perceivers of any phenomenon, we cannot but bring our own subjective categories of knowing to whatever it is we perceive. Although, as Burr (2003) describes, social constructionism is a term that is used almost exclusively in the field of psychology, many of its basic assumptions are also fundamental to sociology. In this, social constructionism has much to offer a relational orientation to coaching, connecting individual experience to the social and organisational contexts in which it arises. Burr (2003) goes on to say that there is no single feature that would identify a social constructionist position, however, it can be loosely thought of as any approach which has at its foundation one or more of the following assumptions originally identified by Gergen (1985).

- A critical stance towards taken-for-granted knowledge. This is about questioning our assumptions of how the world appears to be to us and being critical of the idea that our observations of the world unproblematically and directly offer up its nature and functioning to us.
- Historical and cultural specificity. This refers to the fact that our ways of understanding are historically and culturally specific and undergo evolution over time and in response to events and new cultural trends.
- Knowledge is sustained by social processes. Our ways of deriving knowledge about, and understanding of the world are constructed through our interactions with others.

- Knowledge and social action go together. While there will be a multitude of social constructions of the world, each different construction will determine or invite a different kind of action from individuals. Socially constructed meanings give rise to behaviours connected to those meanings. Thus working to understand meaning and meaning making can give rise to new constructions, which in turn generate new and different behaviours.

In this book we take a primarily social constructionist orientation to exploring how meaning emerges between coach and coachee in a context. We also draw on Western's soul guide and network coach discourses (2017, 2012) as these are highly compatible with an inquiry into the relational dimensions of coaching and the need at times to question taken for granted assumptions about coaching as a profession and its related practices – looking 'awry' (as opposed to attempting to fix or standardise) in order that theoretical and practice vibrancy might be maintained.

An emancipatory ethic

This is not simply an exercise in revealing underlying patterns of thought and meaning, which alone might risk the relativism of certain post-modern perspectives on knowledge, which claim that all points of view are of equal value. Western (2008) points to a particular branch of critical theory rooted in the work of Horkheimer (1987) and Habermas (1971), which is emancipatory in its objectives, challenging the privileging of theory-neutral claims of science and linking these to the values and interests of social groups where the views of the elite are privileged and the less powerful groups are marginalised. Critical theory 'aims to achieve emancipatory goals through revealing and exposing political, cultural and social structures, discourses and practices which impinge on the liberty of individuals and reduce collective agency' (Western, 2008, p. 9). In this book we shall also be taking this stance in relation to surfacing the ways in which wider forces beyond the individual inevitably contribute to shaping lived experience. It is a concern of ours to explore ways in which these dynamics might be surfaced and worked with in service of 'collective and individual autonomy and well being' (p. 9) enabling individuals to grow, while also attending to the contexts and organisations in which they move. In so doing, the possibility emerges of creating conditions through coaching in which dialogue might emerge between individuals about the contexts they contribute to shaping and which simultaneously shape them, in service of mutual flourishing. This inevitably raises ethical questions beyond simply the guaranteeing of no harm to coachees and client organisations, but also in relation to the wider impacts of coaching theory and practice beyond the coaching room. From this perspective, it is no longer possible for coaches to absolve themselves of responsibility as in the familiar coaching dictum 'the coach is responsible for the process and the coachee the outcome'.

Process assumptions and unconscious biases of different theories, social discourses and individuals cannot but contribute to shaping outcomes in particular directions.

Integration

Given the range and breadth of the relational turn, which we cannot hope to do full justice to in this book, integration can provide a meta-model for drawing on a diverse range of theoretical perspectives and paying attention to how these come to inform the orientation and practice of different coaches.

Gilbert and Orlans (2011) set out a number of principles of integration as it has been and is applied in the context of psychotherapy and psychotherapy training. We believe integration offers much for the development of coaches and coaching practice, and is suited to navigating the expanding breadth and depth of coaching theory and the ever-increasing complexities coachees in their contexts are facing. Like social constructionism, integration takes as a fundamental starting point the philosophical position that there can be no one truth. Different theories and approaches (which are social constructions in themselves) will incline individuals to make meaning in particular ways, illuminating aspects of an experience or phenomenon, while also occluding or missing others altogether. This in turn will shape the orientation and specific practices of different coaches. If we take this proposition seriously, then practitioners need to be able to work at the meta-level, be willing to soften any over-attachment to pseudo certainties and hold ambiguities and different starting points. They need to be able to articulate the fundamental philosophical underpinnings of different conceptualisations while also being committed to finding a transparent way through these which creates a coherent form in itself (Gilbert and Orlans, 2011). This is what sets integration apart from 'unaware eclecticism and related fragmented technique' (p. 6). The integrative practitioner needs to be grounded in research-based strategies, which could draw on on a host of different research orientations and work from a 'coherently organized reflexive philosophical and theoretical position within a relational framework' (p. 6).

It seems to us that this proposition has much to offer coaches in navigating the complexities of theory, human relating, development and the contexts in which this is happening. McNamee and Gergen (1999) take a view that any theory is neither intrinsically true nor false. Rather its potential usefulness is revealed through social interaction and processes of negotiating meaning. Theory is not seen as a prescription for social life that is derived from more knowledgeable and objective sources, rather 'a theory is simply a language resource that permits particular forms of action and suppresses others' (p. 5). Such a perspective requires a flexible, contextual orientation as well as 'constant critical analysis, the careful comparison of emerging ideas and theories, and the translation of this process into a coherent set of . . . skills and related process' (Gilbert and Orlans, 2011, p. 6). While this can be demanding for trainers, students and mature practitioners alike, it can also be extremely rewarding and ensure 'constant evaluation of emerging theories and practices, literally a commitment to 'integrity' within the developing professional setting, as well as ongoing critical evaluation of research findings that speak to the potential appropriateness and excellence of service delivery' (p. 6).

What this does not imply is an attempt at uniformity, standardisation or homogeneity of approach. Rather integration offers the possibility of a critically reflective orientation to practice that is aware of the different assumptions embedded in different theories, attempts to find coherence where possible, while engaging with and holding any tensions such as a person centered orientation towards the coachee alongside the results and outcome orientation of coaching in organisational contexts.

Given the ongoing evolution of coaching and the breadth and range of orienta-tions and underpinning theoretical frames that coaches can draw on, integration offers a framework for supporting coaches to develop individual and subtly unique coaching frameworks rooted in contemporary theories of personal growth and development, organisation and systems theory, and wider social and cultural forces which contribute to shaping the profession. It provides a natural evolution beyond the skills- acquisition orientation of much coach training and accreditation. Skills are an indispensable part of professional development, but as professions mature and client situations and contexts become increasingly complex, history shows that there is a need to extend and deepen understanding of the theoretical and philosophical underpinnings behind the deployment of skills. This in turn generates the potential for new and subtler practices to be developed and their impacts researched on an ongoing basis. We liken this to learning a foreign language. Where learning skills is the main vehicle for developing coaches, this is akin to learning language via memorising a series of phrases to be used in different contexts such as ordering a meal or buying a train ticket. This provides a degree of functional competence but will be limited, especially in novel and complex situations. More demanding is learning language by acquiring the components of grammar, syntax, verb conjugations and, over time, the richness of a language's vocabulary, culture and idiomatic expression. This enables the learner to build breadth and depth of understanding as well as skill to communicate situation-by-situation, constructing subtle and nuanced language (coaching) forms as each situation requires, from the simple to the complex and even the poetic!

Gilbert and Orlans (2011) set out a working model of integration comprising the following four dimensions, which we have modified slightly to cater for the context of coaching.

Personal integration

Based on a holistic view of the person, development is seen as being in the direction of becoming more and more integrated and whole. This may involve encountering, surfacing and working with blocks to awareness and the legacy of past experiences that inhibit an individual fully taking charge of his/her life.

It may involve integrating affectively, cognitively, behaviourally, physically and spiritually. Integration is here seen as a model for personal development and growth equally applicable to coach and coachee development.

Integrating theory and practice

This concerns the integration of different theories, concepts and techniques from adult learning theory, coaching-relevant applications of psychology and psychotherapy, coaching as a profession, systems thinking, organisational theory and socio-cultural discourses. It involves drawing together a coherent model of integration from different orientations in the field, which will be unique to each practitioner and guide his or her practice. How a coach makes meaning with clients and deploys particular skills is the embodiment of integration in action. This inevitably involves being sensitive to the different contexts in which coaching is happening, holding perspectives and orthodoxies lightly in order to be able to respond creatively moment by moment and co-construct a coaching engagement with clients that is relevant and meaningful to them and their context. Much coaching literature has been preoccupied with attempting to define coaching and differentiate it from other approaches. A relational and integrative orientation is at once sensitive to existing perspectives at the conceptual level, but also flexible in its practical applications in order to continue to integrate and evolve theory in light of the uses different clients put coaching to and the evolving contexts in which it is being conducted.

Integrating the personal and the professional

This is based on the proposition that the person we are is the coach we are.

This has particular relevance in the context of a relational orientation to coaching where, as will be seen later in Section 2, the unique subjectivities of coach and coachee come together and meaning emerges as these subjectivities interact both explicitly and implicitly. Coach and coachee inevitably impact one another consciously and unconsciously on the basis of life experience, training, beliefs, assumptions, personality style and individual patterns of interaction. This viewing angle presents a radical challenge to the notion of an impartial professional who simply deploys a suite of techniques and expertly 'does to' another. The coach's own internal world, life experience, range and breadth will have a direct bearing on the ways in which he interacts with his clients. This raises the need for coaches to become increasingly aware of their repertoire and range of thinking and action, and be willing to commit to being changed, impacted and developed in the process of being with an other in a coaching relationship. Coaches need to be able to hold the tension between 'false self' or role identity and their 'true self' to avoid a split sense of self when facing the client. This requires coaches to be willing to open to whatever experience is arising in them in the course of working with a client and consider its possible relevance for the work. Coaches also need to be aware of their own limitations, and become aware of blind spots and their own shadow so that this is not projected onto the coachee and the coaching relationship. A need for approval, desire to win more work, wish to be seen to be an expert, and anxiety related to reputation, can all result in coaches subtly and not so subtly exerting pressure on their clients to be and experience what the coach thinks is needed for the coach's own purposes.

Integrating research and practice

This is based on the view of the coach as a researcher of her own work in an ongoing and iterative way. The coach studies research findings and different theoretical frames and integrates these into practice. This includes research from all traditions including quantitative, positivist-empirical as well as qualitative approaches so as not to privilege one over the other but remain open and critically engaged with what each tradition might have to offer. The coach also observes and studies her own practice, paying attention to those factors that facilitate the process of change, personal qualities as well as limitations, and feeds these

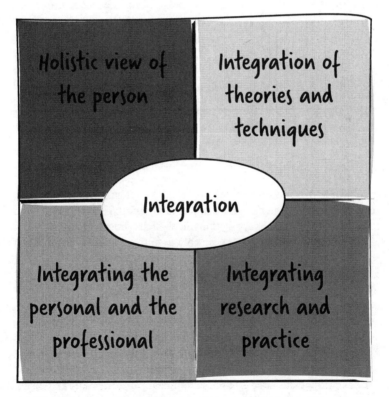

Figure 1.1 The different territories of an integrative approach to coaching

back into her own evolving model of coaching, personal development and research endeavours.

Polarities

A central concept at the heart of an integrative orientation is that of polarities. Polarities are essentially interdependent opposites (Johnson, 1992). These can exist at many different levels in an individual in terms of feelings, thoughts, values, energetic states, preferences, perspectives, points of view and behaviours. At the collective level, different groups can identify with different sides of a polarity in terms of values, processes, ideologies and cultures. Polarities are implicit in what are described as wicked problems, paradoxes or dilemmas, where differing and opposing perspectives and forces are in tension with one another.

Once we open to an intersubjective, socially constructed view of the world, where certainties are less reliable, multiple meanings and differences in perspective have to be negotiated, and individuals have to choose how to respond to ever increasing complexity and uncertainty, the concept of polarities can be a useful orienting framework.

Many writers from different traditions have been interested in the nature of polarities and their role in transformation, learning and development. Jungian theory (Woodman, 1982) posits that creativity arises in the holding of the tension of opposites. Complexity perspectives on organisations point to the need for human systems to hold and be able to work with tensions such as order and chaos (Stacey, 2001). The human relations and psychoanalytic traditions highlight tensions such as communion (joining together) and agency (acting individually), collaboration and competition, leading and following (Hirschhorn, 1998; Vansina, 2008).

Holding polarities in mind

Individualism and positivism, with their roots in scientific objectivity spawn a preoccupation with proving things, with the assumption of objectivity, with right or wrong, setting up binary oppositions in thought. Intersubjectivity and social constructionism call for the need to be able to hold opposite views and different perspectives in mind simultaneously, in relation to one another and in dialogue between people. Rather than prematurely collapsing the tension this creates by leaning towards one end of the polarity and taking up and defending positions, a contextual and intersubjective orientation requires a willingness to consider what each position might have to offer. This is demanding and can be anxiety provoking to the part in all of us that might (especially when anxious) seek comfort in an illusion of certainty with the inevitable preoccupation with right or wrong this gives rise to. Herein lies the temptation of fundamentalist thought.

Polarities or opposites also can guide an integrative orientation to change and development where growth is seen as leaning in the direction of those polarities that are less integrated in the individual or organisation thereby increasing a client's range of responses.

Polarities can exist at the level of thinking, feeling, organisational norms and behaviour, examples include:

Assertiveness–Passivity
Thinking–Feeling
Left Brain–Right Brain
Connection–Separation
Communion–Agency
Grace–Will
Leading–Following
Solutions Focus–Exploration
Surface–Depth
Doing–Being
People–Performance
Relationship Building Interactions–Task Achievement Interactions
Increase Performance–Reduce Cost
Promote Collaboration–Reward Individuals

One developmental trajectory that integration and polarities both point to in the individual is that coaches and coachees need to have access to more range along these continua in order to be receptive, responsive and agile in adjusting optimally to different contexts and situations. A coachee who can only be directive will be less able to listen to his team members and engage them where this might be required. The narrower and more rigid our repertoires, the less flexible we are likely to be in the face of novel, complex challenges and situations. This is equally true for coaches as it is for our coachees.

At the level of interaction between people in a human system, polarity thinking can offer a useful lens for coaching clients who may be experiencing conflict with colleagues in their organisation over what are seen to be fundamental differences. Where these seem unresolvable, it may be that there is a polarity at play. Individuals often hold one position dear and then act out a conflict with those holding the opposite position that appears to be personal or is construed in this way, but is actually based on polarities. This way of thinking can be useful for taking the 'personal' out of interactions and support inquiry, understanding and mediation.

Implications of a relational orientation to coaching and the coaching relationship

The ideas we want to introduce in this book have a number of possible implications for the theory and practice of coaching and the dynamics of the coaching relationship. At its heart coaching remains a conversation-based, one-to-one learning relationship occurring in a particular context (although these ideas also have implications for team coaching, it is not the scope of this book to explore these in detail). The relational turn offers a range of perspectives or viewing angles that cast light on aspects of coaching in particular ways. The following represent a series of emphases that this particular orientation brings to light. It is essentially an orientation with integration at its core, not the learning of a particular protocol or stage model, although these have their place in any individual's personal integrative model.

Core components of a relational orientation to coaching

A relational orientation:

- With its emphasis on intersubjectivity reveals the complex and interactive nature of human systems.
- Is concerned with the self-experience of coachees in their context, how they are impacted by it, make meaning from experience, take up their roles, how they interact with others, and how they are both shaped by and contribute to shaping their environments via the medium of conversations and interactions.
- Is equally concerned with the self-experience of coaches in their professional settings, the different contexts of client organisations and the coaching dyad, how they are at once shaped by and stand to impact clients and their systems.
- Is focused on enabling coachees to respond creatively to ever increasing complexity and uncertainty in themselves and in their contexts.
- Achieves this by enabling coachees to contain anxiety and integrate more and more aspects of themselves, thereby increasing their repertoires for reflection and action all the while acknowledging the relationship between individual and context.
- Makes overt use of subtle and powerful relationship dynamics in the service of meaning making, learning and development.
- Sees the coach's 'use of self' as a central component in facilitating change.

The coach-coachee-context constellation

Fundamental to a relational-integrative orientation and the perspectives offered in this book is a view that coach and coachee come together in a particular context which stands to influence them individually as well as the dynamics of the coaching relationship. Coach and coachee engage in a process of meaning making from their individual experience in relation to one another and the contextual and wider systemic forces that influence and shape them individually and collectively.

The coaching relationship is seen as a two-person psychological system arising in the particular context of a client's organisation, geography, culture and time. Here the minds of coach and coachee are always in interaction with each other and with individuals and forces outside of the coaching room. What arises in the coaching relationship is seen as being contributed to in a host of subtle and not so subtle ways by both participants in their interactions, the influences of the wider field and how these are perceived and responded to. Coach and coachee can never predict precisely how these interactions are likely to impact and influence the feelings, thinking and actions of each. How these interactions unfold simultaneously offers up a rich source of information about the experience of the coachee, the coach, the relationship and the context in which the coaching is happening. A two person orientation requires that coaches work with attention to what each unique client is saying, how he is saying it, what is new or surprising that may not immediately make sense, but is potentially relevant to the client's development, as well as making appropriate use of prior experience and theoretical models. In this respect, every coach-coachee-context constellation is a unique universe to be collaboratively explored. It is in this exploration that new meaning and possibilities for action emerge.

In this book we hope to offer perspectives which may serve to guide coaches and their clients in these explorations. Yet, this is not a book of tools and 'how to do' lists. Rather it is a series of perspectives that might serve to orient those interested in a more expanded and relational view of coaching. Nor can it be any

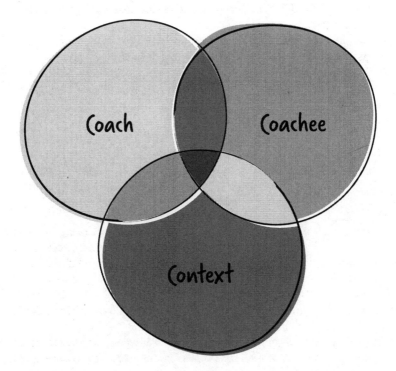

Figure 1.2 The coach-coachee-context constellation

attempt at being a 'definitive' or 'complete' exploration of relational perspectives and their potential contribution to coaching theory and practice. The very essence of a relational orientation means that dialogue and discourse must remain open. Any attempt at pinning down and reducing human experience to a set of exclusive or definitive perspectives is antithetical to the joint projects of integration and relational theory and practice. We believe there is the potential for much further research into the relational dimensions of coaching and hope that the ideas introduced here might act as departure points for further engagement and critical reflection.

How the book is organised

The first section of the book is dedicated to unpacking a series of perspectives on the relational turn that have potential bearing on the theory and practice of coaching. We look particularly at relational perspectives on the self, change and the how individual experience is shaped by context. Section 2 sets out a number of implications of these ideas for coaching practice including a detailed exploration of micro relationship dynamics between coach and coachee. Section 3 explores a number of issues and dynamics encountered in coaching and organisational life that have particular relevance to a relational orientation, or where a relational orientation might offer a wider perspective for negotiating difference and navigating complexity.

We end the book with some of the implications of a relational orientation for ethical practice, supervision and the training of coaches.

Chapter 2

Who is it who is in a coaching relationship?

The question of what 'is' or how do we 'know' and experience the self is one that has long concerned philosophers, psychologists, social scientists, sociologists and more recently neuroscientists. Many perspectives have been put forward to attempt to describe the nature and functioning of the self. All theories (and there are many!) are metaphors, or stories, attempting to describe what is in fact primarily an experience, an experience of being.

It is challenging to write 'about' something that is very experience-near without distancing from the experience. We hope to set out here a number of perspectives on the self that are relevant to a relational orientation to coaching theory and practice, primarily the idea central to relational psychotherapies such as Gestalt (Perls, Hefferline and Goodman, 1951; Philippson, 2001, 2008), intersubjectivity (Orange, 2008; Stolorow and Atwood, 1997), and social constructionism in psychology (Gergen, 2009), of the self and identity as being primarily fluid, socially situated and relational phenomena (Jenkins, 2014). The self as experienced moment by moment, therefore, is seen to be 'always in a process of becoming' (Western, 2012, p. 102), a significant departure from the idea of the self as a permanent, fixed or static phenomenon, which, for Daniel Siegel writing from a neuroscience perspective, 'is actually an illusion that our minds attempt to create' (Siegel, 1999, p. 229).

The relational origins of the self

The individualist traditions and positivist scientific paradigms that have governed investigation into the nature and functioning of the self have tended to portray the self as something that is essentially separate – an individual entity that may interact with others but primarily from a position of separateness and in service of the achievement of individual desires and goals.

Pioneering psychoanalysts like Winnicott (1958,1987; 1965,1984) and Kohut (1984) examined the dynamics of early infant interactions with caregivers and the impacts these have on the forming and functioning of the self. Bowlby (1969; 1973) furthered this work by studying the effect of early attachment experiences on the development of the personality, and highlighted the enduring nature of attachment patterns in adult life. Prior to this, health and maturity had tended to be construed in terms of autonomy and self reliance, with any need for temporary dependence on an other construed as a regression to an infantile state of mind (a perspective which persists to this day in the context of the lonely hero archetype often applied to leaders and leadership). Bowlby's work began to demonstrate that psychological well-being also requires the capacity to make and maintain supportive connections with others, nurture and be nurtured throughout adult life.

Aspects of self-experience

Thinking and the contents of the mind

From a relational perspective, the experienced self can be seen as having both slower moving and more dynamic, rapidly changing aspects. The slower moving aspect of the self comprises the meanings, assumptions, stories, ideas and images individuals have formed about themselves and the world based on early formative interactions with others, attachment, and life experiences to date. It includes values, likes and dislikes, mental models, theoretical and practical learning over the years, and how all of this informs how a person perceives himself, others, the world and how it works. It is also the territory of what in psychoanalytic language is termed object relations (Fairbairn, 1952; Mitchell, 2000). From a relational perspective, our individual sense of self is inseparable from our sense of what is not our self, what is other. As such, our sense of self does not exist in a vacuum but develops in relation to an other. Object relations are particular representations of self-other relationships formed in early childhood, originally with mother or the mothering person of infancy. They are composites of images, thoughts and feelings that give rise to particular motivations and action tendencies. Often unconscious, they nevertheless exert a powerful influence in shaping our sense of self and ways of relating to others and the environment. A coachee may experience a loss of belief in herself and her capability in the face of a boss she experiences as authoritarian, as an object relation of feeling small and insignificant relative to a powerful parent is reactivated in the present moment. An other may struggle to assert his own thoughts and perspectives and believe he has nothing to contribute if he is caught in an object relation formed with a parent experienced as omniscient who told the child what to think and did not support discovery and the child's right to make his own sense of experience.

All of these elements come together to form what can be termed the personality, the unique combination of images and ideas about ourselves and the world that give unique psychological shape to every single one of us and our clients.

We will be aware of some of these elements, while others will be out of conscious awareness, where they nonetheless act as filters determining what we choose to focus on, how we make meaning from experience and choose to act.

One function of coaching is to enable coachees to become aware of those aspects that they are less aware of and which may be visible to the coach and to their colleagues. In this way they can begin to consider whether the way they perceive, think and act is in effect the most accurate and appropriate, given their desires, goals and the challenges and requirements of the contexts they currently find themselves in.

Psychoanalytic theory has demonstrated the ways in which individuals come to identify with mental content and representations and take them to be who they are (Mahler, Pine and Bergman 1975; 2000). In this way a sense of identity or ego is established which confers a degree of familiarity, consistency and predictability in relation to who a person knows himself to be and how he believes things work or should work in the world. Different individuals identify with varying degrees of attachment and rigidity. Someone who is very identified with the belief 'I don't like foreign food', formed on the basis of past negative experiences, may not be inclined to try *any* flavours that are unfamiliar, thereby denying themselves the possibilities of new and potentially pleasurable experiences among the vast array of new taste opportunities.

Similarly, a leader may be strongly wedded to beliefs about the importance of hierarchy and command and control as being the only legitimate and appropriate way to achieve organisational effectiveness and personal success. His identity might be fused with images of being authoritative, potent and controlling of the environment. As such, he may struggle to adjust and develop the skills and behaviours necessary to negotiate and co-construct meaning and strategy where multiple stakeholders with different subjectivities and perspectives may need to participate in this process.

Identification means that we experientially take ourselves, often unconsciously, to *be* the images and beliefs that we hold about ourselves. This is one of the reasons why change can be difficult. In changing a core belief, relaxing identi-fication with a particular self-image and opening to the implications of a very different worldview to one we have held for a long time, we undergo a change in our very sense of identity. The leader in the example above, finding his familiar way of seeing himself and operating in the world challenged by the context he finds himself in, may experience confusion and disorientation as his familiar strategies, attachments and resulting identity fail to have the impact he desires. To the extent that as individuals we identify with our beliefs and mental content is the extent to which this can feel, from the perspective of the ego, like a psychological death, which in turn can generate much anxiety and resistance.

Understanding this dimension of the self is increasingly relevant in the context of coaching individuals who, faced with complexity, may need to question their deep-seated beliefs, attachments to particular roles, assumptions, strategies and identities in order to develop greater agility, more effective and creative ways for responding to their organisational challenges.

Feeling and the body

As human beings we are not, however, in our direct lived experience, simply a collection of past experiences and the self-images, stories and mental representations we have formed from these. We are also somatic beings with bodies that experience sensations and emotion. Moment by moment our bodies are a rich source of information about how we are experiencing ourselves, sensing the wider field, the dynamics of different contexts we are in, and constructing meaning and our participation in the world. Body oriented practitioners and researchers from a range of disciplines have shown that mind and body are not split as in the Cartesian fallacy of 'I think therefore I am', but are part of a whole, where feelings and thoughts reciprocally influence one another and are inextricably linked to the wider context in which an individual is situated (Damasio, 2006; Kepner, 1999, 2003; Kurtz, 1990; Ogden *et al.* 2006; Strozzi-Heckler, 2014). Furthermore, the beliefs about ourselves and the behaviour they give rise to, through repetition become encoded in body posture, movement tendencies and tension holding patterns (Frank, 2001).

Many of us will be familiar with the sense of energised, expansive lightness that often accompanies the experience of delight or joy, or the muscular contraction and tight chested fluttering that accompanies moments of anxiety. As we become more and more sensitised to our bodies and the information they hold, coaches and coachees can learn to tune in to ever more subtle states which can offer up much valuable information about how we are constructing our sense of self, our current reality and experiencing ourselves and the environment we find ourselves in. Our sensations and emotions are also the territory of intuition. Porges's (2011) research into the role and functioning of the vagus nerve, which conveys sensory information about the body's organs to the central nervous system, has demonstrated a sound neurobiological basis for the experience of 'gut feel' as a form of reliable knowing. One role of an integrative and relational approach to coaching is to enable coachees to become more aware of, and able to think about, the information offered via their bodies, which often bypasses some of the conscious and familiar content of the personality. This can be a more accurate reflection of a coachee's and coach's experience and patterns of being in the world than their mental constructs alone. It is interesting to note that the word 'mente' in Italian, meaning the 'mind' has the same etymological root as the verb 'mentire', meaning to 'lie'.

Cultivating greater body sensitivity is not without its challenges. In Western cultures there has been a tendency to privilege rationality and the mind over the body (Hamill, 2013; Strozzi-Heckler, 2014). We tend to privilege the experience we have of ourselves as being able to 'think' our way through life, constructing stories about our experience in language, thinking in linear, causal and deterministic ways about how to be or how to function, and imposing these constructs onto any experience. Neuroscience research has revealed that prior to our conscious capacity to notice what we want or want to do, our brains will already have processed vast amounts of sensory input and begun to orientate towards a particular action (Damasio, 2000).

Lehrer (2009) describes that our initial and immediate reactions, including twinges of feeling, are the distillation of details that are not perceived consciously and that much of what we think is in fact driven by our emotions. He goes on to say that 'in this sense every feeling is really a summary of data, a visceral response to all of the information that can't be accessed directly . . . feelings are often an accurate shortcut, a concise expression of experience' (p. 29). This has significant implications for coaches and coachees navigating the complexities of the VUCA world where reason and logic alone may not provide sufficient information for examining responses to what is complex and unpredictable in order to create a viable response or course of action. Opening to sensations and being able to think about the meaning they contain increases the ability of coaches and coachees to perceive more of what might be contributing to a current situation or problem, and support greater creativity and imagination in response. Lehrer (2009) reminds us that 'the process of thinking requires feeling, for our feelings are what let us understand all the information that we can't currently comprehend. Reason without emotion is impotent' (p. 31).

Body oriented approaches to development and change (Kurtz, 1990; Gendlin, 1997) have long appreciated the transformative and creative value in suspending mental constructs and turning awareness to bodily felt experience, while temporarily relaxing attachment to mental content, an orientation which is also at the heart of the Gestalt approach (Clemmens and Bursztyn, 2003; Kepner, 1990) and mindfulness practices (Hall, 2013; Kabat-Zinn, 2004).

Human development, in particular our capacity, formed in early months and years, to regulate arousal and manage our inner state is critical here. Coachees (and coaches) who have not developed the capacity to bear uncertainty, novelty or complexity may either drop into rigidity of thought, flat energy, or experience anxiety, confusion and feelings that are experienced as overwhelming. We shall explore the need to regulate the nervous system in Section 2.

Being able to sense into feeling states is fundamental in being able to read human interactions and sense the quality of a culture, meeting or team climate. This is also key to coaches being able to open to their own body sensations as a source of information about the coachee, the coaching relationship and the context in which the work is happening. Where coaches can work in this way, notice what is arising in their bodily experience, this can inform interventions in ways that are sensitive to what might need paying attention to but might not yet be obvious at the level of thought and conscious interaction (Francis, 2005). This is at the heart of making use of oneself as an instrument of change (Rainey Tolbert and Hanafin, 2006) and reading the dynamics of every unique coach-coachee-context constellation. Conversely, some people can identify with emotions alone, as if they are the primary source of reliable information and act on this basis, with little or no thought and reflection. One important function of coaching is to help clients develop the capacity to experience and make sense of feelings, emotions and bodily intelligence in the service of effective thinking, meaning making, relating and action required to navigate the VUCA environment successfully.

Taking action

Another key element which contributes to describing how we experience ourselves in the world is the capacity we have to make choices about what we want to achieve, how we want to go about having our needs met and fulfilling our desires through taking action. This is our ability to identify what we intend, our purpose, or what a particular situation requires from us. This then focuses our attention and efforts in particular ways and directions in order to respond to what is required, or influence the environment where we can in order to achieve our objectives. This capacity involves identification of needs, intention, selection of options, focus, choice and the de-selection of other possibilities and actions that are not in keeping with our primary intention or objective in that moment. It is also the aspect of ourselves that can take those actions necessary for our well-being and effectiveness. Existential and Gestalt perspectives emphasise this capacity to take action and engage in the world and its importance in conferring meaning and well-being (Perls, Hefferline and Goodman 1951). Knowing what we want and what matters to us is central to knowing who we are, having a mind of our own, and is at the heart of Western's (2017, 2012) Soul Guide discourse.

These three dimensions of thinking, feeling and taking action, which make up the lived experience of the self, do not exist in isolation but in relationship to one another. They also influence one another and inform the choices an individual makes, how he behaves in the world and responds to individual needs and those of the organisation/context he finds himself in. Early experiences shape beliefs, the ability to regulate anxiety and the capacity individuals feel they have when faced with novel or challenging situations. These patterns reveal themselves in the context of the coaching relationship.

A coachee may be physically exhausted and close to burnout as a result of overwork. She may be aware of her body feeling permanently fatigued and anxious given the pressures of the environment and how she is responding. She may have 'out of awareness' or untested beliefs that she should be able to do everything that is required, that if she is not superhuman she will be seen as weak. As a result she may believe that she cannot afford to stop and take care of herself. This could generate increased anxiety every time she is faced with the fact that she has more on her agenda than it is humanly possible to do. Unless the belief can be surfaced, her attachment to it understood, tested, and anxiety regulated, it is possible that she will continue to try harder, risking more serious consequences to health and professional performance such as burnout (Cassereley and Megginson, 2009). She will not be able to orientate herself in a way that is appropriate to her need for rest and more balance while also attending to that which needs to be done and finding ways to adjust to that which cannot be.

Another coachee comes wanting to work on being more assertive in a way appropriate to his role. He becomes aware that he has a belief that assertiveness is close to aggression and that he believes aggression is bad. He comes to see that being liked is important to him and confers a sense of security. The prospect of not being liked gives rise to a tightness in his chest and racing heart. As he senses into this tightness he realises that he has an assumption, based on past experiences, that if you do not make too many demands on people, they will like you. He has a strong belief that assertiveness is likely to turn people against you. As the coach explores with him the nature of these beliefs and what it might mean for the client to risk occasionally not being liked by some if a situation calls for decisive, authoritative action, the client starts to feel anxious. This coach suggests a supportive experiment in the form of mindfulness and breathing exercises to see if these might enable the client to regulate down the intensity of his physiological anxiety. He describes a reduction in stress, and in time, as he practices reducing anxiety, and increasingly trusts in his ability to do so, he is able to experiment with incrementally more assertive behaviours which had hitherto been experienced as too risky and, therefore, unavailable to him in his repertoire as a leader.

Co-emerging selves – A dynamic relational perspective

So far we have described the dimensions of thinking, feeling and taking action, and how they interact and mutually influence one another in the organism that is the person of the coach and coachee. We hope that the lived experience underpinning each of these categories has been, at least in part, recognisable. We now want to go one step further to suggest that experientially, the self can be thought about as the direct experience we have of ourselves moment by moment as we interact with the world and those in it. While this moment-by-moment experience is happening in all interactions, it also serves as a framework for paying close attention to the dynamics between coach and coachee and the interactions each has with others in the client context. This is a radical departure from the modernist individualistic conceptualisation of the self as closed and separate, striving for autonomy and primarily acting upon the world. Instead, the relational self is rooted in perspectives from the post-modern era and seen as more fluid and provisional, rather than fixed and enduring (Izod, 2008), where the individual is seen to be as much shaped by the world as being a participant in shaping it.

Gestalt writers (Perls, Hefferline and Goodman, 1951; Philippson, 2001, 2008) have long considered the self not as something internal to the individual, but actually located at the boundary between the organism and the environment. Malcolm Parlett (1991) emphasises this in describing individuals and their experiencing as always being situated in a context or wider field: 'The essence of field theory is that a holistic perspective towards the person extends to include environment, the social world, organisations, culture. The more assiduously we can navigate with the various field theory maps, the more we are likely actually to perceive and recognize the indivisibility of people from their surroundings and life situations' (p. 70).

Neuroscience and infant research have amply demonstrated that we are constantly constructing our experience of ourselves in relation to the environment (Cozolino, 2010; Beebe *et al.*, 2005; Beebe, 2000; Stern, 1985). In the context of coaching this supports the notion of a coach-coachee-context constellation where the experience of all participants is being shaped by relational interactions and forces at work in the wider field. This also resonates with complexity perspectives on organisational life where patterns of thought, knowledge and behaviour arise through the interaction of different systems in a particular context. Cavanagh (2006) uses a metaphor of water to describe this process. The components of the phenomenon that is water are H2O molecules, but whether what we see is ice, steam or snow depends on the relationship between the molecules and the environment. The attachment patterns, personality, meanings and skills an individual has formed over the years will emerge, recede and interact differently with one another in different contexts, with different challenges, environments and relationships, including the coach-coachee relationship dyad. Thus the self (of coach and coachee), in a host of subtle and not so subtle ways, is likely to appear and be experienced differently moment-by-moment and context-by context. From this perspective the coach can be thought of rather like an anthropologist who inquires and invites his clients to inquire into the unique dynamics of each coach-coachee-context constellation for what they may have to reveal about the co-created patterns between coachee and context, coach and context and coach and coachee.

We are constantly having to respond to our individual needs and aspirations in the context of being connected to one another and the world around us. A coachee's needs and goals arise from the interplay of his individual history, meanings, intentions, relational templates and the requirements of stakeholders and the organisation context. The ever-changing external environment is constantly placing demands and expectations on us and our clients that we might not be able to anticipate or predict, and yet need to be able to respond to in every unique coach-coachee-context constellation. How we experience these requirements and how we respond given the interaction of thinking, feeling and taking action constitutes the moment-by-moment dynamic flow of individual experience, the dynamic self, and is a central focus of inquiry in a relational orientation to coaching.

Beliefs and cognition for both coach and coachee arise in response to what is happening in the environment and can colour and shape how phenomena are experienced and made sense of as they are apprehended by the sensory systems of the body. Sensations, movements and actions are simultaneously coloured by and shape these meanings. It is the interplay of cognition, perception, sensation, emotion and movement which all contribute to how each of us organises our experience in the present moment in relation to the context we find ourselves in.

A leader may hold dear values of inclusion and engagement and be very committed in a work context to listening and allowing her team members to express their views about strategy, implementation and the co-creation of appropriate and aligned behaviours. She may be less inclined to assert her own views and lead from a hierarchical position. When oriented toward inclusion she may appear relaxed, open and receptive. Her tone of voice and conversational pattern may be measured, curious and inviting of dialogue. When a crisis arises, the field conditions change and, as a result of her team looking for guidance, and the situation calling for quick and decisive action, she may find herself issuing clear direction and instruction, with little or no engagement of others. Her body may appear more tight and compact, her movements more staccato, and her tone of voice clear, strong and definite. This leader's ability to respond fluidly depends on her range and flexibility along the facilitation – direction continuum, willingness and skill to act in a different way that is more suited to the requirements of context, and the ability to read the field conditions to determine what might be required.

This potential for flexibility demonstrates what Gergen (2009) refers to as a repertoire of selves, embracing the fact that we become subtly and not so subtly, different versions of ourselves moment by moment and from context to context. This is also true of coaches in our relationships with different clients.

Over time we all develop familiar patterns of thinking, feeling and responding to the environment (with corresponding skills and behavioural repertoires that become more and more finely honed and automatic as we practice them). As has been seen, these familiar patterns can offer a sense of coherence and continuity, but can also become limiting or narrow repertoires that are not always going to be fit for purpose given the novel challenges we and our clients face. In fact, any meaningful change is likely to involve a re-organisation of these familiar patterns and expansion beyond 'comfort zones'. Not all coachees (and coaches) will necessarily be able to respond to the requirements of shifting contexts with ease and fluidity. They may not yet have developed the meaning making and practical skills required, or may have out of awareness beliefs and assumptions inhibiting them from experimenting with acting differently. These often become apparent when inquiring with clients into how they are responding to and making sense of their current situation. Coaching can support clients to increase in awareness and the necessary range of skill and capability to read the field conditions, make informed meanings, evaluate options and respond in timely and effective ways to uncertainty, complexity and novel situations.

The patterns of interaction that coach and coachee enact together also offer a rich potential source of information about coach and coachee self-experience and meaning making, yielding much learning if they are inquired into. It is this inquiry that is at the heart of a relational orientation to coaching where the primary focus is on enabling clients to expand in awareness range and flexibility for responding to ever increasing complexity in their contexts. This approach to developing the capacity in clients for 'creative adjustment', central to the Gestalt approach (Sichera, 2003), is particularly useful in the context of the VUCA world.

Most people will be able to identify a significant difference in their experience of themselves when on a relaxing holiday as opposed to being at work and about to participate in their annual appraisal conversation with their line manager. While these significantly different contexts are useful for illustrative purposes, each of us, every moment of every day, will be experiencing subtle shifts in energy, posture, thought processes, focus, comfort, discomfort, dissatisfaction, satisfaction speech and behaviour. All of us organise ourselves in relation to the environment on the basis of what we are encountering 'out there' and the workings and interplay of thinking, feeling and the choices we make 'in here'.

Authenticity

The notion of a more fluid self-experience can be a challenge to assumptions of an essential 'core' or authentic self that have emerged from the self-actualisation drive of Maslow (1954) and still persist to this day. Here there can be an implication that the self is some kind of object, a permanent quality or thing to be aspired towards or uncovered. It can also become confused with beliefs and self-images an individual is identified with and which need to be maintained for a sense of coherence. From a more relational perspective of a fluid and shifting self-experience this is problematic. Existential philosophy offers a way of thinking about authenticity that is more accommodating of a conceptualisation of the self that is fluid, contextual and relational. From an existential perspective, authenticity as described by Sartre (1956; 1997) involves an individual confronting reality, including all its shadows and challenges, facing up to it without regret and assuming responsibility for his or her actions. As such, authenticity is not a fixed or essential quality of a person that remains static, but is a quality that arises on the basis of an individual choosing authentic responses to whatever situation she finds herself in. Although challenging, this can be a useful and liberating notion for coachees facing increased uncertainty and complexity, and where past models, behaviours or protocols are no longer adequate. It opens up the possibility for coaches and coachees to relax striving to find the 'right' answer where no single perfect response is available, and explore and consider the current situation, evaluate options and identify what the coachee is willing to commit to authentically and in good faith.

The present moment

In working with a relational orientation to the self in coaching it is useful to consider how we structure time. In many relational orientations great emphasis is placed on the present moment and this will be explored further in subsequent chapters. In relation to our discussion of the self, it is important to stress that the self is always being organised in the present (Stern, 2004). In fact, the present is all there ever is. The future may be imagined in the present, but once it has arrived, it is no longer future but becomes the present. In imagining a future, it is inevitable that motivations and patterns of expectation and anticipation formed in the past also come into play in the present moment of imagining. The past may be remembered, but remembering is still happening in the present moment. Research into memory has shown that what is remembered is actually being created and re-created based on stimuli that are occurring in the present and that how events and experiences are re-membered (put together again) can be different every time (Schore, A. 2003; Siegel, 1999). In the present moment, therefore, our self experience may contain aspirations for the future that has not yet arrived, and patterns of thought and behaviour shaped by past experiences as remembered, as well as those patterns of thinking, feeling and behaviour that have formed over time in the past and influence how we currently experience ourselves, the world and make meaning. In a coaching conversation, coaches and coachees simultaneously need to pay attention and respond to whatever is arising in the present in their individual experience, between them, in relation to the context in which they are working and to the stated objectives of the work (imagined future). How the present is made sense of and is responded to, along with expectations and hopes for the future, create the dynamic in which change can occur. This present moment focus can be challenging for coaches who have been schooled in a more solutions and future focused orientation. Yet simultaneously managing the demands and dynamics of the present also supports shaping an emerging future by influencing and re-working patterns of thinking, feeling and acting. The precise ways in which the future may arrive can never be fully known in advance. In this way, exploring the ways in which a client constructs his self experience stands to facilitate the expansion of repertoires beyond those familiar patterns that may be ineffective or limiting in relation to the challenges and development goals of the client. A particular implication here is that what is imagined or constructed as desirable at the start of a coaching intervention may not be what actually becomes the focus, or where a client ends up. This can be challenging to the linear and mechanistic logic which often governs a primarily goal oriented approach to coaching. Opening to an intersubjective approach allows the possibility that the construction of goals can itself also be explored on an ongoing basis, in order to decide if what is imagined at the start is actually what might be required for meaningful and context-relevant development to occur. It is therefore important to continue to review experience in relation to stated objectives throughout the coaching process. We do not mean to imply here that goals are not important, but wish to suggest that they may need to be held lightly enough for meanings to be clarified and new and potentially more appropriate possibilities to emerge where appropriate (see David, Megginson and Clutterbuck, 2013 for a comprehensive exploration of the nature, role, benefits and challenges of goals in contemporary coaching theories).

Example

A coachee came to coaching with an overt and expressed need to improve his capacity to manage poor performance in his team. This objective was also supported by his line manager. With his coach he described feeling stuck and simultaneously anxious in relation to this development objective. Rather than moving quickly into imagining a future where he was able to manage performance well, the coach asked the coachee if he would be willing to explore both the experience of stuckness and the feeling of anxiety as they were making themselves felt in the moment. By using a two-chair technique familiar to Gestalt practitioners, the coach invited the coachee to sit alternately in one chair representing his anxiety, and the other chair representing his stuckness, and simply report on what he experienced in each. The coach encouraged and supported the coachee to see if he could bracket off any pre-suppositions or internal self-conscious voices and open simply to experiencing, in the present moment, whatever was arising for him in the form of sensations, feelings and thoughts. In the 'anxiety chair' the coachee described feeling his heart racing and a tightness in his chest. His boss then came to mind, and he spoke of fearing that he would be judged harshly if he were unable to turn around the performance of his team in a short time. He went on to talk about not knowing how to proceed. In his frustration and anxiety he had developed a tendency to bark orders at his team, further alienating his reports. He believed he had exhausted his existing repertoire and did not know what to do, this in turn, made him feel more anxious. He then moved to the 'stuckness chair' and his demeanor changed. He appeared initially to relax a little and reported that here his heart was not beating so fast. When asked to sense into the experience of stuckness without judgement or evaluation, he reported that he felt pinned to the spot, he did not know where to turn. As he described this he then reported that his chest had started to feel tight again. When asked if there was a thought associated with his tight chest he replied 'It's not OK not to know and be stuck'. The coach, aware of the interplay between cognition and sensation, and feeling a contraction in his own chest as the client spoke out his belief about not knowing, then wondered aloud whether this specific thought might be contributing to his anxiety and interfering with the coachee's ability to experience the stuckness. He gently suggested to the client that he might, if willing, try to experiment with dropping the thought and come back to the direct sensation, in the present moment, of stuckness and being pinned to the spot. At this, the client went on to describe how there was some sense of peace in not being able to act. He could just sit and wait. His coach encouraged him to describe in as much detail the felt experience of peace As he made more room and space in himself to sit with and experience directly the relaxing aspects of not having to do anything, the coachee began to be able to think differently about his challenges and reflect more deeply on the motivation and personalities of team members. He also became aware of the cultural forces at play that had contributed to years of poor performance being tolerated in his part of the business. Over time this generated a host of different conversations and strategies for addressing the poor performance of his team.

This coachee was organising his experience in a particular way in relation to his challenge. Anxiety and stuckness, as a result of feeling pressure to perform (reinforced by the outcome orientation and drive of the dominant managerial discourse in his organisation), and the meanings he was attributing to this experience, were maintaining a self-organisation where he was unable to think differently or creatively in relation to the challenges he faced. By studying closely his experience and identifying how his patterns of self-organisation were working in the here and now, how they were causing anxiety and unhelpful stress, and by being able to regulate this down with the help of his coach, new possibilities began to emerge. As we become aware of existing patterns of thought, feeling and action, and experience their impacts directly with awareness, they can relax and make room for new patterns to emerge that might be more useful. From a neuroscience perspective, exploring and feeling the nature of current patterns through focusing on different aspects of how clients are organising themselves in the present moment, allows familiar neural firing patterns to be interrupted and new neural networks to be formed (Azmatullah, 2013). These mechanisms and processes will be unpacked further in later chapters.

Development and emergence of the self

From a relational perspective the experience of the self arises moment by moment at the boundary between the organism and environment. New experiences and the complexity of the VUCA environment challenge the existing beliefs and ideas of both coaches and coachees about how best to proceed. Both are called upon to reflect on their experience and thinking in the moment, the dynamics of the situation they find themselves in and generate, often new, possibilities for response and action. This process is developmental in that in increasing the capacity to respond creatively, coachees and coaches also stand to increase in awareness, skill, range and repertoire. These processes are often at work in the context of transformational coaching and organisation development such as that set out by Fisher, Torbert and Rooke (2003), which draws on the work of constructivist-developmental psychologists such as Susanne Cook-Greuter (2004), Jane Loevinger (1987) and Robert Kegan (1982). Here, it is the need to respond to the novel and that which is disorienting that acts as a spur to the development of new meanings, perceptions and identities.

Practice implications and interventions

Viewing the self and the experience we have of ourselves moment by moment as intimately connected to others, the context we are in, and how we are responding, has a number of important implications for coaching practice such as:

•   Exploring how the coachee perceives and organises himself in relation to his context and its dynamics. This includes attention to the ways in which coachee and context are co-constructing identity, role and action.

- Exploring how the coachee organises herself in, influences and is influenced by, significant relationships, and how these patterns might be changed where necessary in order for new, more optimal, possibilities to emerge. Importantly, this includes attending to how supported and resourced coachees are in different relationships and how able they are to access support where necessary.
- Exploring how coachee and coach mutually and reciprocally influence one another in the coaching conversation. How the coach experiences herself, if seen as influenced by context, will simultaneously hold information about the coach, coachee, their relationship and wider contextual forces at work.
- Noticing automatic repeating patterns as they arise in the present, thereby increasing awareness and allowing more choice to become available.
- Experimenting with new patterns of self-organisation and action.
- Inquiring into how the coaching intervention itself is being co-constructed in each coach-coachee-context constellation via the interplay of different organisations of meaning among participants and stakeholders.

In terms of role, the coach provides an 'other' to whom the coachee can speak. Western (2012) points to the centrality of speaking in relationship to the formation of the self where speaking 'in a coaching session is to speak oneself into existence' (p. 150). This is also attested to by the etymological roots 'per sonum' (Latin for 'through sound') of the word 'persona' meaning person or personality. How the coachee speaks, what he speaks about, and the effect this has on the coach are rich sources of information about the coachee and his constructions of self and reality which may only surface to conscious awareness in the speaking and interaction with the 'other' of the coach.

Coaching informed by the model of the self as set out here can enable clients to explore the ways they currently organise themselves, relax familiar patterns and experiment with different ways of self-organising that are better suited to the challenges and demands of whatever situation they find themselves in. Malcolm Parlett (2000; 2015), writing from within the Gestalt tradition, has described five 'abilities' that can support greater creativity and agility in the face of complex, uncertain and ever changing contexts these are:

- Responding – The ability to organise ourselves to do what might optimally be required in response to different situations we encounter. This includes initiating, adapting, compromising, leading, following, doing nothing, stopping doing something.
- Interrelating – The ability to relate effectively one to one, in groups and communities, including dealing creatively with differences and conflict.
- Self-recognising – The ability to be aware of what we are doing as we are doing it, making sense of our experiences, lives and purpose and being alert to our capabilities, development needs and limitations.

- Embodying – The ability to experience ourselves as visceral, physical beings, opening to the sensations and the 'feeling' of what is, and being able to be touched and impacted at a fully human feeling level. It includes being able to express who we are moment by moment with all of our being emotionally, physically, energetically as well as intellectually.
- Experimenting – The ability to explore whatever possibilities and opportunities are present and being willing to question and change self-limiting ways of thinking or repetitive patterns that may have outgrown their usefulness.

Cultivating awareness of the dynamic and relational nature of the self along with the capacities outlined above develops in individuals access to what Parlett (2015) describes as 'whole intelligence' including cognition as well as sensation and intuition. It stands to equip coaches and coachees with the resources necessary to navigate the complexities of their situations on an ongoing basis and beyond the time frame of a particular coaching intervention.

Chapter 3

Relational coaching and change

Two distinct and interrelated approaches to change

The linear causal model is (nevertheless) very useful as long as one is aware of its limitations and never forgets that this kind of linear cause-and-effect relationship does not actually exist, but is our way of simplifying a much more complex reality.

Compernolle (2007, p. 39)

The client is not a problem to be solved or a story to be listened to. The client's present experience is a vivid example of how all experiences are organised and is an opportunity to study how and why experience gets organised in just that way.

Kurtz (2008, p. 12)

Compare the following two vignettes and consider what each might be saying about the coach's implicit assumptions about change.

I

A client comes to coaching with a clearly stated intention to work on developing leadership presence and gravitas following an appraisal which identified that, while a technical expert, the client lacked the experience required to lead his team through a period of strategic change. The coach takes time at the start to explore what having leadership presence and gravitas would look like for the client. The client says he imagines this to involve feeling more confident and being able to direct the activities of his team clearly. The coach contracts with the client to work in this direction. The coach then designs a series of exercises to enable the client to achieve his stated objectives of being more confident and developing the capacity to communicate more powerfully. The coach suggests a series of voice and speech exercises, along with posture and breath work to enable the client to experience himself differently and take up his authority in the room with the coach. Initially the client seems a little reluctant but, with encouragement, is soon experimenting in the room with different behaviour. Occasionally the client seems a little flat and begins to talk about how challenging he finds his role and that, at times, he can doubt if he has leadership potential or wants the role. At this, the coach reminds the client that he has no doubt the client can achieve his stated objectives and steers the client back to practicing the tools to support greater embodied presence. The coach is alert to when the client might 'drift' from the original contract and is quick to remind the client what they have contracted for, ensuring they remain focused on the original objectives. When the client reports back that he was not able to act on his learning and agreed experiments in a meeting between coaching sessions, the coach is quick to remind the client of the contract they have between them and with stakeholders. He holds him to account for not having followed through and encourages him to persevere and simply try out the new behaviour, for that is how change will happen. Whenever the client appears to be low in energy, the coach becomes more energetic in an attempt to transmit positivity to the client. When this fails, the coach suggests an exercise in listing all the positive attributes the client has to draw on. The coaching comes to an end and the client reports that the exercises were useful in enabling him to see what was required to be a leader in the new situation he faces. He reports that he has made some changes and verbally commits to continuing to practice the skills he has acquired.

2

The same client comes with the same development agenda. When the client talks of his challenges, the coach is struck by the apparent lack of energy in the client. Initially she keeps this to herself as she does not yet feel she has the rapport with the client to support her making a direct observation. She focuses instead on asking questions about the client's role and context and how he is currently experiencing his relationship to his role and team. She concentrates on being as present to herself and the client as possible. The client talks energetically of past roles and successes and his love of the technical aspects of his role. She senses some mild anxiety and stage fright in herself and has a tentative thought that the client might be struggling to know how to be in this new situation and is anxious about the development feedback he has been given by the organisation. She notices in herself that this mirrors a slight anxiety she feels in the face of not yet knowing how best to support the client as it is still early days in their relationship and she is not up to speed with the context. She decides to make a number of empathic interventions and, informed by her feelings and tentative meaning making, says aloud how challenging it can be to expand from being a technical expert to being a strategic leader of others. She adds, from her own experience, that although this is a challenge it can be rewarding, but she and the client have yet to discover together what might be possible for the client to achieve in the time they have available. At this point the client seems initially to relax and then says, 'but I only have six sessions with you!' The coach notices a slight contraction in her chest and fluttering in her solar plexus and associates this with feeling with the client the pressure he is under to get a specific result in a short amount of time. She intervenes with a comment that it is unlikely that the client will have developed everything he needs to be a leader in six sessions, but that her hope is that they would be able to get some foundations in place by the end to support his on-going learning. She adds that one of the enemies to their working effectively together might actually be the idea that they need to get somewhere specific and get somewhere fast, even though this is an understandable and familiar pressure in organisational life. Developing leadership presence, she goes on to say, could be thought about as a never-ending project.

When the client talks about self-doubt, and failing to put his learning into practice, the coach normalises this as inevitable when we are on the threshold of learning something new. She wonders and explores with the client whether what he challenged himself to achieve might have been a little too far out of his comfort zone and how they might co-create an experiment that is sufficiently stretching and realistic given the client's levels of resilience. The coach continues to explore the client's reality in relation to the situation he finds himself in, including the expressed need to become more authoritative. Her emphasis is on working to really understand the client's situation as he experiences it and constructs it in his mind, and communicating this understanding as best she can through words, energy and tone of voice, letting the client experience how she is being impacted by his story. During this conversation, the client becomes aware of thoughts and concerns that are getting in the way of his acting with more authority, he surfaces a number of limiting beliefs. As he lets himself see the part he is playing in holding himself back he reports beginning to feel, think and act differently in the organisation. He reports that he is experiencing an increase in energy and more support and resilience in himself to continue to develop.

These two vignettes are written in an intentionally polarised way to illustrate how two distinct orientations to change might look in practice. The first is written to illustrate an approach to change steeped in assumptions from the individualist, rationalist and modernist traditions and can be summarised as linear. The second reflects an orientation informed by more recent relational and post-modern ideas, which can be summarised as emergent. Both have their place, and different clients may respond differently to each. From an integrative perspective we want to explore different ways of thinking about change to enable coaches to develop range and be able to calibrate their practice appropriately to different coachee personalities, situations and contexts.

Modernist and linear approaches

A linear approach to change is based on assumptions of causality and a belief in there being a series of laws which underpin human experience and development rooted in traditions such as positivism, Newtonian physics and individualism (Wheeler, 2000). These approaches, concerned as they are with discovering laws, processes and mechanisms that underpin how the natural world functions, assume that these laws can be used to predict cause and effect and inform interventions designed to bring about change in particular ways by following a series of steps. They sit comfortably with a construction of coaching as a vehicle for getting from a current state to a desired end state. From a neuroscience perspective, this approach makes use primarily of 'top down' processing where the prefrontal cortex is used to direct learning in particular ways, inhibit certain sensations, and where cognition and intention are harnessed to guide focus and activity (Cozolino, 2013; Ogden *et al.*, 2006). Coaching theory and practice that is rooted in these assumptions is more likely to be characterised by hard behavioural goals, contracts, processes and procedures and a deterministic view of change, where the coach's role as change agent is to act on the client through questioning and technique to bring about development. A coach standing firm in this orientation to change is likely to be informed by a protocol based approach. He will offer exercises and structured approaches to exploration and experimentation with an end in mind. The coach may act as a gatekeeper, adhering more closely to assumptions and beliefs about change, and challenging behaviour in the client which does not fit with the coach's working assumptions about what needs to happen to enable the client to achieve his or her stated goals and arrive at a solution. This approach to change will seek to identify what needs to change, take necessary action to close the gap between the current state and desired 'end' state. It is often characterised by doing. The primary focus is on what has been agreed is needed and how to get there as efficiently as possible. There is a focus on outcomes as the main event, and relating is considered important only in so much as it can facilitate the achievement of specified outcomes. Energetically there is more of an emphasis on will as the driving force for change (Denham-Vaughan, 2005).

Post-modern and emergent approaches

This approach to thinking about and facilitating change is not so invested in assumptions about linear causality. Instead, the assumptions here are more informed by relational, post-modern ideas, and those from quantum physics and complexity (Mindell, 2000). While there is an assumption that there is some reality 'out there', the meaning it is invested with, how it is understood, engaged with and responded to is a complex process involving multiple possible perspectives and subjectivities. How we look at the world and ourselves, the assumptions and schemas we bring, determine what we see and what we bring into being as our particular version of reality. This includes our sense of our own capacity and capabilities in the contexts in which we live and work. While there is an assumption that experiences and phenomena are interconnected and do influence one another, simple linear cause and effect logic is expanded to include a belief in complexity and the inter-connectedness of multiple factors giving rise to whatever is being observed or experienced. Where a coachee might be feeling anxious about a presentation, a primarily individualist and linear orientation might focus on how a client can develop and practice the skills involved in designing and delivering a successful presentation in order to overcome anxiety through mastery. A more emergent and post-modern orientation would be more inclined to lead the coach to be interested in the uniqueness of each coachee's experience of anxiety and the complex web of factors that might be giving rise to it in both the coachee and in relation to the context in which he is working and at that moment. Coach and coachee might explore together how the coachee's organisation of experience is giving rise to anxiety in the present moment with the coach, and what might support regulation in the here and now. The coach would then be interested in studying with the coachee the impact of any change occurring in the present moment on his orientation to preparing for and giving presentations.

There are now many examples that demonstrate the interconnectedness of field conditions and the feelings, thoughts and behaviours they give rise to. Dire consequences have been linked to behaviours resulting from the interaction of particular complex field forces and the human agents impacted by them as in the case of the Mid Staffordshire Health Trust in the United Kingdom (Francis, 2013) and the Challenger shuttle disaster in the US (Schwartz, 1990). Here the failure of individuals to consider the impact of system forces and anxiety on patterns of human interaction, decision-making and behaviour, and attempts to control and achieve specific outcomes, rather than inquire into and consider the complexities of organisational life, contributed to situations where individuals lost their lives.

With an emergent orientation, the emphasis is more on accepting and exploring what is arising in the present moment and in the relationship field of the coach-coachee-context constellation. The focus here is on exploring in depth the coachee's organisation of experience, how she makes meaning and constructs reality, paying attention to the interplay between the individual and her context. Sensations, feelings as well as cognitions are treated as having equal potential value and relevance in support of discovery and meaning making. From a neuroscience perspective this orientation can be seen to be more oriented towards 'bottom up' processing (Ogden *et al.*, 2006). The focus is on sensations and present moment experiencing. Insight and articulation of meaning emerges from this experience in interaction with the coach. Meanings and assumptions are held lightly and reflected on critically, rather than simply being imposed on the basis of a pre-determined set of assumptions. This approach supports more the integration of feeling, thinking and action as opposed to the acquisition of a particular set of skills alone.

The coaching contract offers a degree of bounding and focus for the coaching work, but in this orientation to change, it is held lightly, defining the territory in which there is also freedom to explore, where outcomes and unexpected developments arise from being in an exploratory relationship. Attention to specific goal achievement is balanced with abiding in the present moment and allowing more what is present to emerge and be considered. This is particularly suited to complex situations and tricky problems, where there are no clear solutions or outcomes to be aimed for and where coachees need to be able to hold the tension of competing forces and identify the next best step to take. As such, outcomes may also differ from that which was originally identified, but can become more relevant and appropriate to the client and context as more of the total situation will have been considered. Resulting behaviours are also likely to be more realistic and sustainable, as there will be more support in the client for new behaviour to be experimented with. Energetically there is a surrendering to what is and to grace (Denham-Vaughan, 2005).

Gestalt perspectives on change reflect this more relational and emergent orientation to change and this is summarised in Beisser's (1970) paradoxical theory of change. Here change is seen to happen naturally when we stop striving to be something we are not currently, but fully experience what is. This perspective on change draws on Aritstotle's notion of 'physis' (Clarkson and Cavicchia, 2014) that the human organism is naturally oriented towards growth, development and wholeness (Perls, Hefferline and Goodman, 1951). What is required for change to happen here is to fully connect with and experience the ways in which an individual is currently organising his experience of himself and the environment, including current and familiar patterns that may not be optimal. The principle of 'enantiodromia' going back to Heraclitus (Waterfield, 2000) is also useful here. It was taken up by Jung (Samuels, 1985) and is implicated in the theory of polarities as used in the Gestalt tradition (Joyce and Sills, 2014). Here the assumption is that when any force becomes too strong or abundant then its opposite will arise. This gives rise to the counterintuitive (in a linear paradigm) practice of amplifying and experiencing directly what is, including resistance and stuckness, in order for something to move and for change to happen.

Implicit in this way of working is a belief in an individual's capacity for self-regulation and balance and that the individual will re-organise in the direction of health and growth providing enough relevant information about the current situation is brought into awareness (Wollants, 2007). This will inevitably also surface the ways in which someone is inhibiting their natural drive towards growth and development.

Working with limitations to change

The ways in which we can limit our potential for growth are many and include beliefs we have developed about ourselves and the world based on past experiences and the meaning maps or 'schemas' we have made from these. This is also the territory of procedural learning, the familiar and habitual ways we respond to the world that have become encoded as quick-firing neural pathways and corresponding sensations, movements and resistances (Ogden et al., 2006). Much of these processes and how they work is out of conscious awareness. It is inevitable that as we turn our attention to how we and our clients organise our experience of ourselves moment by moment, we come to see a host of familiar patterns that hitherto had not necessarily been in our conscious awareness.

This allows the possibility for these patterns to be evaluated and their current usefulness in relation to our development appraised. It is likely that these patterns will have some usefulness and relevance in particular contexts and situations. They become problematic when they become fixed responses that limit our creativity and response-ability in relation to novelty and the learning required in the face of new challenges. Action learning (Torbert, 2004), and reflective practices such as double- and triple loop learning (Tosey, Visser and Saunders, 2011), which invite clients to surface their assumptions, evaluate their effectiveness and develop alternative assumptions and strategies, are well suited to this way of thinking about change.

Different clients will respond differently to the two orientations to change set out here. We see both as having a role in facilitating change while also being different and emphasising different aspects of the change process. The Boston Change Process Study Group (2010) stress that for change to occur it needs to happen in both the declarative or conscious verbal domain (of which the linear, logical conscious interactions of coaches and coachees are part), as well as the implicit procedural or relational domain, which is the territory of feeling, rapport and how the client feels welcomed and met in relation to the coach. We shall expand on this in Section 2.

If we see linear and emergent as two opposites on a continuum, it is important for coaches to develop the range and flexibility to move along the continuum in response to what the total situation of client preferences, issues and context dynamics, including other stakeholders, might require in every unique coach-coachee-context constellation. Having access to both orientations is also useful for situations where in the early stages it appears that coachee and stakeholders are aligned around shared objectives that seem to be understood consciously and conceptually, and the coachee seems motivated to make the identified changes, but where it then becomes apparent that all is not what it seems. In spite, initially, of apparent motivation, as the coachee begins to grasp what actually may be required, she may find it difficult to make necessary changes, revealing in the privacy of the coaching conversation different needs and motivations than those stated publicly at the start with stakeholders. In situations like these it may be crucial to the effectiveness of the intervention to be able to move from an initially linear orientation to a more emergent one. In this way more of the underlying assumptions, meanings and dynamics, both personal and contextual that might be making it difficult for the coachee to take action can be surfaced. This then creates the possibility of reframing the coaching intervention and offering opportunities for more meaningful and realistic change to occur for the client that is also sufficiently appropriate for the context in which the work is happening.

Mindful awareness

In order to activate the developmental potential of paying close attention to how we and our clients construct ourselves and our realities in the present moment, a particular quality of attention is required, that of mindful awareness. Mindfulness based approaches to change have been gaining in popularity in psychology and coaching over the last ten years (Boyatzis *et al.*, 2005; Chaskalson, 2011; Gilbert, 2009; Hall, 2003; Kabat Zinn, 2004; Siegel, 2010). It will be clear to many readers that awareness itself is not always sufficient to facilitate change. Many of us know what we need or even want to do in order to feel better, develop new skills, experiment with new possibilities, yet many good intentions can lead to little appropriate or sustained action.

Mindfulness is the capacity to observe ourselves moment by moment without judgement. As we practice mindfulness-based observation our capacity for awareness becomes more and more sophisticated and subtle. We experience an increased intimacy with ourselves and our experiencing and it is this intimacy that supports change to occur.

The neuroscience of mindfulness

How can something so apparently simple, counterintuitive from a linear and deterministic perspective, and so lacking in future orientation and striving facilitate change? For a perspective on this it is necessary to turn to the growing body of neuroscience research in this area (Gilbert *et al.*, 2008; Hölzel *et al.*, 2011; Lutz *et al.*, 2004; 2008). Syed Azmatullah (2013) cites a study conducted in Toronto where two groups of adults were studied in relation to a mindfulness-based stress reduction programme. One group was trained in mindfulness-based stress reduction techniques over an eight-week period, while the other group was wait-listed for the training to take place after the study. Both groups were asked to engage in either a narrative focused activity by considering, for example, what a personality trait adjective meant to them, or an experientially focused activity sensing their body state without purpose or goal, tracking and noticing any changes from moment to moment. Subjects were scanned in an MRI scanner to see which areas of the brain were most active during the various exercises.

The narrative focused activity was associated with much brain activity in central midline brain areas, whereas the experientially focused activity was associated with much activity in more lateral (outer, side areas) areas of the cortex. Of note is that in those not yet mindfulness trained, this lateral activity was particularly concentrated on the left side, where task-focused activities are normally performed. Mindfulness training shifted these patterns so that experientially focused activity in mindfulness-trained subjects was associated with more activity in the right cortical areas, the insula and somatosensory areas. This indicates that mindfulness training seems to change the connections in the brain so that narrative story telling that ascribes preconceived meaning to sensations is reduced, enabling us to experience sensations directly (Farb *et al.*, 2007). These results, along with other studies (Crane, 2008; Ogden, 2009), have shown that mindfulness training results in structural changes in connection pathways and that the change is long lasting. The stronger the connections to brain sensory areas, the more we are able to experience sensations directly without the automatic association of preconceived meaning formed in the past and connected to the sensation. This includes all the out of awareness beliefs, assumptions and justifications that create immunity to change as described by Keegan and Lahey (2009). In mindfulness practice, every time we notice our mind wandering into narrative generation, we are encouraged to simply notice this and redirect attention back to our sensation. Repeatedly doing this builds up neural pathways, strengthening connections to sensory brain areas rather than those connections to areas of the brain associated with self-referential, repetitive story telling. In this way, anxieties and stress associated with such stories are alleviated. Relief from stress and anxieties promotes an improved mood and sense of well-being and significantly affects mental processing, increasing capacity for reflection, problem solving, experimentation and choice of action. This seems to confirm from a neuroscience perspective what Beisser (1970) was pointing to, based on experience and observation, that simply noticing and experiencing without automatic meaning making facilitates the relaxation of familiar patterns of self-organisation and the emergence of new patterns of thinking, feeling and action. There is also much evidence that positive mood and outlook is one of the most significant factors associated with optimal functioning, growth, resilience and flexibility (Fredrickson and Losada, 2005 cited in Azmatullah, 2013). Positive outlook and affect have also been seen to be fundamental to high performance in business teams (Losada and Heaphy, 2004 cited in Azmatullah, 2013).

The interruption of automatic, preconceived meaning making on the basis of sensations is fundamental in enabling old constructions of self, what we might think we are or are not capable of doing and what we imagine the consequences of new action to be, to relax. It also supports the relaxation of attachments to prior knowledge and biases. This relaxation of familiar meaning schemas and narratives and their corresponding feeling states, postures and behaviours allows for the possibility of old beliefs and identifications to be appraised and new versions of self and action strategies to come into being, so necessary for responding in complex, ambiguous and uncertain contexts. Rather than knowing ourselves from the 'top down', the past meanings we hold about ourselves in the cortex which then might influence the feelings we have and actions we take, we now have the opportunity to suspend these beliefs and experience ourselves from the 'bottom up'. Feeling and observing our sensations without judgement allows for old patterns of expectation and anxiety to be appraised in light of present moment direct experience. In this way new meanings and self-images can be made and old beliefs expanded upon, updated or re-written if necessary.

Being able to sense our bodies and tune into the subtlety of our experience without judgement is key. Fritz Perls (1969) one of the founders of Gestalt therapy was on to this when he issued the invitation to 'lose your mind and come to your senses', recognising that recounting narratives about our histories risks reactivating over and over familiar patterns of thought and reinforcing the status quo. By making more room for sensation and tracking the flow of sensation in the body, we open to a rich territory of experience that can relax familiar patterning in the brain hence 'lose your mind'. The statement 'come to your senses' conveys the need to learn to attune more to the body and experience without judgement. It also points to the fact that in doing so we actually come to 'sense' meaning both sensation and greater mental health, well being, creativity and richer, expanded meaning frameworks for living and working well, increasingly able to respond to complexity and novelty.

Perls (Perls *et al.*, 1951) is also credited with describing anxiety as 'unsupported excitement'. Neuroscience is now confirming the reasoning based on close observation behind this assertion. The direct experiential reality of anxiety and excitement are very similar. We might feel a knot in our stomach and tightness in our chest along with a raised heartbeat (Porges, 2011). It is all too easy for many of us to label these sensations as anxiety based on past experiences and narratives we have constructed as a result. These sensations often arise in conjunction with an experience of something new, different and challenging. If all we can do is see and understand these sensations on the basis of preconceptions about risk and exposure, we are unlikely to be able to find the support and resources in ourselves and the environment to stay with new experiences, or those which take us out of our 'comfort zone' long enough for learning, experimentation and growth to take place. What converts the same sensations from associations of anxiety to associations of excitement is the ability to suspend familiar meaning making as happens with mindfulness practice, and find support in self and the environment, including the coach as in the second example at the start of this chapter.

A coach worked for a number of years with a series of senior leadership teams in a multinational organisation. Her role was to provide team coaching and process consultation as the teams worked to develop strategies and system interventions to be able to respond in an agile way to a series of never ending challenges and complex problems in both the internal and external environment. The dominant culture of the organisation was positivist and rationalist and as such meetings tended to be very tightly managed with extremely full agendas, information sharing and little or no time for exploration, reflection, collaborative meaning making and experimenting with new behaviours. A frequent result was that agendas were never satisfactorily worked through, leading to frustration and feelings of failure among many team members. Over time the coach noticed a particular pattern that captured her attention. Frequently conversation would drift from a particular agenda item with its implicit focus on problem solving and arriving at a quick solution. This was in part due to the issues being complex and affecting all members in different ways. When this happened the energy in the room would tend to become more animated and alive, and individuals would speak from the first person, sharing their own perspectives and surfacing more of the underlying complexities they faced. This would continue for some time until one of the group (and this was often a different member in each team every time) in the face of no solution immediately presenting itself, would say 'we are going down a rat hole – let's get back to the agenda'. At this, conversation would stop and the team would usually agree to hand the problem to a working party to be taken off line. Occasionally this would result in a resolution, but more often than not the issue would return at the next meeting and a similar pattern would be played out. The coach saw this happen over a number of months and reflected in supervision on its repetitive nature. She speculated with her supervisor on what it might have to say about familiar processes and cultural patterns in the organisation in particular an apparent inability to sit with and tolerate the complexity, uncertainty and messiness of human relating that was more unpredictable than the teams were used to. Shortly afterwards the coach was attending another meeting where the conversation was becoming more animated and unclear. At the point at which one of the team said 'we are going down a rat hole' she heard herself say 'how do you know this rat hole isn't a potential tunnel out of your familiar stuckness and inaction?'

There was a moment of silence and, thanks to the coach having a trusting relationship with the team, they were able to explore how they might change their conversation patterns to allow more space for reflection, for listening to one another and considering the different perspectives on the problems they faced. Over time they experimented together with naming, normalising and containing anxiety long enough for different conversations and new possibilities to emerge. Individuals were able to express that the 'rat hole' statement had come to be used as code for 'we are frustrated and anxious that we don't seem to be getting anywhere on this issue so let's move on'. The team also had not yet developed the capacity for generative dialogue and tended to advocate and defend different positions, further contributing to a lack of cooperation and progress. Over time team members developed the understanding, skill and self awareness to listen more to one another and use difference to generate options which they then were able to commit to and align around as a result of everyone feeling heard and included, even where not all agreed personally with a particular option for action.

Whenever we are on the edge of a new development or expansion beyond the familiar we are likely to feel a mixture of both anxiety and excitement – anxiety based on past meanings and the fact that we are often facing into the unknown, and excitement at the potential for discovery, novelty and growth contained therein.

Coaches can be a powerful resource for clients in enabling them to develop the mindful awareness of existing patterns and the support needed for growth and change to occur. Coaches have a role in enabling clients to contain and regulate anxiety so that they are sufficiently stimulated for learning to occur but not so anxious that learning and experimentation are inhibited. Coaches also need to be able to track their own experience mindfully to access their own creativity. When as practitioners we find ourselves, for whatever reason, in the grip of anxiety, we can resort to familiar patterns (usually in the form of intervention protocols or random questioning) or control in order to feel safer, but the cost of this is a contraction of the space for new insight and possibility to emerge.

Let us return to the client example at the start of this chapter.

The client came to coaching with a clearly stated intention to work on developing leadership presence and gravitas following an appraisal which identified that, while a technical expert, the client was seen to lack the experience required to lead his team through a period of strategic change. The coach has taken time to set out her way of working and has gained permission at least in principle from the client to pause occasionally to check how the client is experiencing and constructing his experience in the present moment.

By now the coachee has begun to identify for himself what having leadership presence and gravitas might involve for him personally and he seems energised and committed in relation to developing greater confidence and ability to set clear strategy and vision, drawing on the different skills and experience of his team members. The coach has taken time to explain her way of working and some of the science behind a present-moment mindful orientation, which appealed to the technical expert part of the coachee who seemed interested in understanding more. The coachee has also developed greater sensitivity to his body as a source of information about how he is organising his experience in relation to his challenges. At this point coach and coachee have been talking about a forthcoming team meeting where the coachee is intending to experiment with different behaviours. As he talks about this the coach notices the coachee's levels of energy dropping and his voice becoming quieter.

COACH: *As you speak you seem to be losing some of the energy you had earlier and your voice is becoming softer, are you aware of that?*
COACHEE: *Now that you mention it yes . . . I am losing my enthusiasm.*
COACH: *What are you experiencing as you notice a loss in enthusiasm?*
COACHEE: *I feel my shoulders are getting heavy and my mind feels sluggish all of a sudden.*
COACH: *Would you be willing to sense into the feeling of heaviness? What is it like?*
COACHEE: *It feels like a pressure, pushing me down?*
COACH: *. . . and when you notice that pressure, pushing you down, how does it affect you?*
COACHEE: *I feel a bit flat and helpless . . . it's not good is it?!*
COACH: *Would you be willing to suspend for a moment the judgement that it is not good and simply stay a little longer with the sensation of feeling flat and helpless to see what might happen next, if you just stay close to the sensation?*

Client looks a little hesitant but seems to relax on hearing the coach's supportive and encouraging tone of voice.

COACHEE: *I can try. I am not used to just staying with things. I normally just get on with things, get busy.*
COACH: *Are you feeling a pull to get busy now?*
COACHEE: *Yes, I am feeling frustrated.*

COACH: *So getting busy is a familiar pattern of yours?*

COACHEE: *Yes.*

COACH: *So we have an opportunity to slow down moving to the familiar pattern and see if anything else shows up that might be of use to you. Are you still feeling frustrated?*

COACHEE: *Yes.*

COACH: *How does frustration feel to you right now?*

COACHEE: *Like a tension in my arms and chest.*

COACH: *Feel into that tension and see if there is a thought that goes with that feeling.*

COACHEE: *. . . I think I should be able to do this.*

COACH: *Do what?*

COACHEE: *I should be able to lead this team, set the pace and let them get on with it; they are all experienced after all.*

COACH: *And as you have that thought?*

COACHEE: *I feel more tightness and some anxiety.*

COACH: *So when you think you should be able to lead the team and let them get on with it, you feel more tightness and anxiety?*

COACHEE: *Mainly when I think 'let them get on with it'.*

COACH: *So you mainly feel more tightness when you think let them get on with it?*

At one level this might appear to be a simple paraphrasing statement but it is also designed to support the client to stay close to his experience in the present moment and points to the relationship between sensation and cognition.

COACHEE: *Yes, I am not used to delegating. I have always been a doer and in control.*

COACH: *So I imagine it is new for you to be in a situation where you have to let others do more?*

COACHEE: *Yes. It is new.*

At this point the coach notices a subtle drop in the coachee's tense shoulders, which have been frozen for some time. The coachee's face relaxes slightly.

COACH: *What happened when you let yourself see that this is a new situation for you?*

COACHEE: *I felt a little relief. My shoulders feel a little more relaxed. Like it is not up to me to have to do it all.*

CLIENT: *How does it feel to see that?*

COACHEE: *I feel a mixture of relief and still a little anxiety.*

Coach and coachee were able to see that a familiar pattern for the coachee of organising himself was to have the belief that he should be able to it all (as had actually been the case in his former role where he was a subject matter expert and where others relied on and frequently sought his advice). Faced with a change in role and less control, given organisational and team complexities, he initially felt a loss of identity and motivation in the coaching for stepping up to the challenges. By studying closely in the here and now how the client was constructing his experience through the interaction of thoughts, feelings and sensations, the client was able to see how his familiar pattern of control was inhibiting him in orienting to the new challenges where he was facing into the unknown and could not, therefore, predict outcomes. Also he was struggling with trusting his team and delegating. Over time the coachee also became aware of a series of beliefs not only to do with being in control, but with also needing to be seen to know what to do. As more and more of these underlying beliefs and their corresponding feeling states and behaviours were surfaced and explored in the coaching relationship, the coachee began to discover more room for the possibility of occasionally not knowing and for trusting more in the clear capability of some of his team members to know enough. He was able to feel more resourced and relaxed in the face of uncertainty as he had more and more experiences of being able to work things out together with his team. Over time he began to develop a sense of himself and identity as a facilitator of his team's effectiveness, which did not mean having to know it all, but required the ability to set parameters and then work in dialogue to harness the different talents of his team and ensure alignment with overall strategic objectives.

Working in this way requires coaches to be able to trust in the process of the coaching relationship, its reciprocal gestures and responses, and bear moments of uncertainty in themselves and in their clients. Understanding the mechanisms involved here can be important. This can be challenging in that it appears to run counter to the dominant culture of fast pace and quick fixes found in many organisations. Where coaches can integrate more of a present moment focus in to their work, the benefits for coachees can be great and much learning and growth happens in a short period of time. Conversations can become deeper and interventions more subtle and impacting. Not least because coaches can relax a tendency to keep asking coachees what they 'want to do' or 'could do' as in a primarily solutions focused orientation. Coachees in the process of working something out in a complex situation can feel assaulted by this line of questioning, as if they should quickly be able to identify a strategy. Instead, they can be supported to explore themselves, their context and the interplay between the two, and generate new strategies more rooted in the subtleties and complexities of their personalities and total situation. It is this experience of learning and transformation that communicates to clients the value of this orientation. It is not an orientation that can easily be described or 'sold'. It needs to be experienced directly.

Linear and emergent perspectives on change both orientate coach and coachee in particular ways facilitative of change. If either is overplayed it is likely to reveal its particular limitations. In practice coaches need to hold a tension between linear and emergent approaches, moving between them on the basis of the particular contours of the coach-coachee-context constellation in which they find themselves. Given the dominance of a linear orientation to change in the managerial discourse (Western, 2012) of many organisations, coaches need to be able to meet their clients and the sponsors of coaching initially in the orientation that is familiar to them. Over time, as trust builds in the relationship and/or circumstances dictate, coaches may then be able to find ways to move between a linear or more structured orientation and emergent approaches that might better serve the learning agendas of coachees and the complexities of their organisations.

Comparison of strengths and challenges of each orientation

Type of Approach	Strengths	Challenges
Linear	Can be focused. Good for short-term work. Suited to relatively simple development agendas and contexts. Easier to 'sell'. Aligned with dominant striving outcome and solution orientation, so experienced as familiar.	Narrow and constraining the field of possibility. Can feel pressured and manipulative. Can objectify the client – risk of subject-object relating. Overly simplistic. Hierarchical and expert driven. Preoccupation with being right or having 'the way'. Literal.
Emergent	Relational. Deepens reflection skills. Suited to discovery. Making new meaning. Suited to complex situations and development agendas. No predetermined attachment to the 'right way', instead openness to discovering what makes sense to the coachee in context moment by moment. Emphasis on meaning making. Can feel freer. More democratic where questions of power can be surfaced. Leverages the implicit relational and is embodied. Sees resistance as multi directional energy to be explored.	Can drift and lose focus without skill on the part of the coach in facilitating the coachee's meaning making. Requires maturity and skill on the part of the coach to track closely what is unfolding with the coachee. Requires self-awareness in the coach and capacity to bear uncertainty. Can be hard for clients to see the value of this approach ahead of experiencing it, as it is counter-intuitive to a dominant striving for solutions orientation.

Chapter 4

Selves in context

Navigating and negotiating organisational life

Each of us comes into, and has to interact throughout life with, a world that is full of pre-existing meanings and familiar and established patterns of thinking, interaction, expectation and norms. These make up the very culture of a society and any form of human system for that matter, be it a group of friends, club, school, church or organisation. Each family system, or equivalent, into which children are born, will have a unique quality and dynamic between members, children and attachment figures, as well as reflecting to a greater or lesser extent the norms and patterns of the society and time in which it exists. From the very beginning each child's 'organisation of perceptions, feelings, purposes and operating strategies is also influenced by the ideas which exist independently of the relationship, such as principles of child rearing, the beliefs and prescriptions of a society' (Marris, 1996, p. 66).

Thus the meanings we hold and those held by others are central to how we organise our experience. At the heart of this process is how we experience, and negotiate for, ourselves in relation to different meanings, discover how we relate to them, select what we choose to identify with, align with and hold dear, or evaluate and reject. As Marris (1996) points out 'we cannot say anything about what this 'I' is or wants which does not become a statement about the way experience has been organized into a structure of meaning regulating behaviour' (p. 33).

The relationship between the uniqueness of individual experience and fitting in with pre-existing meanings and narratives gives rise to a fundamental polarity inextricably bound up with the experience of a relational self, that of experiencing oneself as being similar to or different from – 'me' and 'not me'. In relation to communities and organisations, this polarity underlies the dynamics of agreeing and disagreeing, belonging or standing apart, joining with or separating from, cooperating or asserting a difference.

Relational templates

Early relational experiences with caregivers establish templates for relating that persist into adulthood where they continue to shape perception and interaction often out of conscious awareness. These templates become highly significant in organisational life particularly where individuals have to build relationship networks and make meaning together in the service of the success of the enterprise.

In optimal parenting, with just the right balance for the child between responsiveness to his or her needs, containment and regulation of anxiety, a child experiences being able to connect with others, yield to support, take it in and be nourished by it. With enough space also for exploration and autonomy (for example being allowed to make simple decisions, at times, such as what to wear) a child develops a sense of personal will, separateness and agency. For many of our clients, and for us as coaches, early experiences were not optimal and can leave us ambivalent, anxious and resistant in the face of either connecting with or standing apart.

Winnicott (1957) demonstrated how the comings and goings of caregivers has a profound impact on the developing mind of children, a perspective that is increasingly being confirmed by relational neuroscience (Cozolino, 2006, 2010). At times, the quality of a parent's energetic presence and touch can be experienced by the infant as an impingement, intrusive and overwhelming. Similarly, absences can be experienced as too long and abandoning. These experiences directly affect the biological development of the brain (Teicher et al., 2004) and disturb the infant's felt sense of coherence and ultimately the meanings he or she creates about his or her safety in the world (Porges, 2001).

With sufficient experiences such as these, infants fail to develop an enduring and coherent sense of self and experience the boundary between them and the world as fragile. Changes in the external environment are then experienced as threatening and anxiety provoking. Bowlby's (1969, 1973) work on attachment demonstrates how inconsistent parenting interferes with the development of a 'secure base', an enduring sense of physical and emotional consistency and safety. With a secure base adults are able to confront novelty, differences and difficulties without becoming too disoriented or distressed. They are also able to contain higher levels of anxiety and nervous system arousal, go on reflecting on their experience and consciously choose their responses rather than reacting on the basis of anxiety and defensiveness. We shall explore this particular perspective further in Section 2.

This has clear implications for building and maintaining relationships at work and developing the skills necessary for inquiry, dialogue and meaning making (De Haan, 2012). Individuals with a secure base are more likely to have the ability to move fluidly between joining and autonomy, connection and withdrawal, and to know that both options remain available as different situations require. Less secure clients may project a critical parent image on to a manager or the organisation and manage this either in the form of unquestioning compliance or reactive rebellion. Nevis et al. (2003) have identified the importance of balancing both intimate and strategic interactions in organisational life. Intimate interactions are any human interaction where the primary focus is on enhancing closeness between individuals. Strategic interactions are any interaction where the primary focus is on the achievement of an organisational task or goal. For organisational effectiveness, they argue, both these types of interaction need to be woven together as a 'seamless braid'. This will depend on individuals' capacity to both be positively impacted by connection and human support as well as tolerate a reduction in this supportive connection in order to get on with task activity.

Another tension here is that human systems, societies and organisations all need to develop common or shared meanings and understandings to which individuals need to subscribe in order to function smoothly and confer some sense of order, predictability and a reduction in anxiety. By the same token Marris (1996) stresses that 'because each of us has loved, uniquely, these parents, this mate or child or friend, and so has experienced, wanted what no one else has wanted, and learned our own way of making sense, common languages always distort and inhibit what we can express, organising the world less sensitively to our particular attachments' (p. 82). This tension is also true of coaching theory and the evolving identity of the profession where membership to different coaching bodies hinges on allegiance to established protocols and approaches, and where individual professional identities, preferences and thought might be lost in group identification.

This points to a fundamental dilemma faced by each of us as coaches and as clients when we have to find ways to manage ourselves, with one another, and in the organisational and societal contexts in which we and our clients find ourselves working – the need for security and belonging in predictability, *common* languages, assumptions and meanings, and the need to have our *individual experiential uniqueness* acknowledged and allowed degrees of expression. From the perspective of individual and organisational learning and change, exploring different subjectivities and constructions relative to dominant and enduring patterns of meaning and behaviour is also key to transformation and innovation, and yet it can be difficult to do.

Relational templates formed in early interactions with caregivers can be reactivated in relationships at work (Krantz, 1993; Pooley, 2006.) Individuals can be acutely sensitive to the potential for their uniqueness to be somehow negated, impinged upon or dismissed. They may either hold back from asserting their difference or assert it so forcefully and stridently that it results in alienating their audience, such as in organisation meetings which are characterised by individual posturing, advocacy and defending of positions (Cavicchia, 2009). Systems of patterned and enduring thinking resist questioning because the individuals who subscribe to them can thereby avoid the personal anxiety that comes with an acknowledgement that what is thought of as known, knowable, predictable and safe is, in fact, more accurately a construction that is temporary, partial and changeable.

This tension experienced at the individual level can also be seen to operate at different levels in teams and communities. At the organisation level it is seen as the tension between sameness, structure, predictability, control, on the one hand, and difference, flexibility, uncertainty, emergence on the other. Coaching from a relational perspective frequently involves exploring how the coachee is experiencing and managing this tension and, with some clients, such as those who might be perceived to be mavericks by other members of the organisation, is often central to the work of coaching itself. It also has a major bearing on learning in organisations of which coaching is just one strategy.

Writers from a wide range of traditions all consider that difference and novelty are the source of new learning and meanings, especially given the view that we cannot solve intractable problems without new learning (Gant and Agazarian, 2005; Laloux, 2014; Stacey *et al.*, 2000). Given the complexities of organisational challenges and human systems, first order change (concerned with performance improvement via the application of existing knowledge) is proving to be limited. Increasingly there is a need to expand into second and third order change. The former is concerned with surfacing and evaluating the strategies and working assumptions behind current approaches, the latter with questioning and experimenting with different paradigms and working assumptions as situations require (Watzalwick *et al.*, 2011). From the field of constructivist-developmental psychology, development in adults involves expanding perspectives, meaning making capacities and the ability to navigate a world that, unlike in earlier stages of development, is no longer thought of as primarily controllable through the exercise of existing expert knowledge, power or will alone (Cook-Greuter, 2004; Fisher *et al.*, 2003; Kegan, 1982). Thus complexity and novelty can catalyse development in the individual and the individual's responses also stand to influence the context, although precisely how cannot ever be fully predicted.

Individuals in any social system or context are faced with a series of personal tensions. On the one hand, how much to join with the prevailing ideology, culture and norms of the context, thereby experiencing belonging and potentially compromising their sense of autonomy and individuality. On the other, how much to question or stand separate and apart, thereby asserting their difference and potentially compromising their sense of belonging (and risking ejection if this difference is too marked). This is particularly relevant to coaching leaders faced with complex challenges in a VUCA environment.

One of the central foci for exploration and collaborative inquiry in a relational orientation to coaching is what happens for individuals in their context. How do the context and dominant ways of working inform their sense of self and their thinking? How do they experience the requirements of their role and situation? How does an individual manage the boundary between his or her sense of personal self and role identity? How does this then give rise to the particular ways in which an individual organises him or herself in response? To what extent does this self-organisation support health and growth while balancing individual needs and organisation requirements?

Sameness and difference – attention to coach and coachee positions in relation to context

Gestalt psychology (Philippson, 2001) and relational theories of the self (Bromberg, 1996; Gergen, 2009) are concerned with the multitude of possible versions we might construct of ourselves in relationship to the ever-shifting field of the environment and individual needs, and how we manage the tension between needing a sense of coherence in how we experience ourselves as well as opening to the potential to be far more fluid in our responses than we might think we are (Bachkirova, 2011). This can be a particularly helpful perspective where coach and coachee have to negotiate their own differences, meaning making and possibilities for action in the context of the organisation and wider society in which the coaching is happening (Cavicchia, 2009). In Gestalt theory, the concept of the 'contact boundary' between organism and environment captures this dynamic whereby individuals need to develop a sense of personal boundary that is permeable enough to take in nourishment and connection with the environment, but also sufficiently impermeable to reject that which is experienced as overly destabilising, toxic or too alien to be assimilated (Mann, 2010).

An easy way to collapse these tensions when contracting for coaching is to adopt the view that he who pays the piper calls the tune, aligning primarily with the organisation that is paying for the coaching intervention. Yet this reductionism, while creating an illusion of reduced complexity and a working 'solution', is not without its challenges. Jennifer Cock (2010) describes how the guiding principle of 'do no harm' so enshrined in much coaching theory is problematic. By aligning primarily with satisfying the requirements of context, coaches risk harming their clients by denying them a mind of their own. By 'mind of their own' we are not suggesting a mind isolated from context, but the experience of being able to explore and think about themselves in relation to context and choose how they might wish to respond, as opposed to a stance of blind allegiance to the ortho-doxies of a particular culture. Conversely, by aligning more with the coachee's world and concentrating on meeting individual needs, coaches risk harming the organisation by discounting the role requirements, culture and dynamics of the organisational field. This polarisation risks encouraging a climate of either compliance (where the individual suppresses difference and merges with the environment) or defiance (where the individual asserts difference in order to stand separate from the environment) in clients and, judging by the experience of many supervisees, in coaches too! These positions can be conscious choices, but when polarised, are all too often out-of-awareness reactions based on unexamined early relational patterning. One possibility which thinking in this way provides for coaches and coachees is that they can reduce the automatic nature of unexamined patterns and increase range, choice and flexibility for moving along the continuum of merger and separateness. This stands to support more dialogue between individual perspectives on a situation or challenge and the current ways these are being thought about and responded to in an organisation.

In Figure 4.1a, individual and organisation are disconnected. The boundary between the coachee and the organisation is rigidly impermeable allowing for nothing of the organisation to cross over and influence the coachee and vice versa. This may be as a result of the individual fearing a loss of autonomy and as a result tightly defending his or her position and separateness. Although

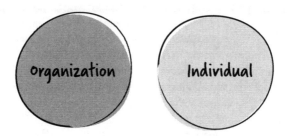

Figure 4.1a Individual and organisation disconnected – impermeable boundaries

differentiation between individual and organisation is high, there will be little or no dialogue and learning and the potential for conflict will be high. A coach operating from this position might over-privilege the coachee's experience and needs and discount the requirements of the organisation.

In Figure 4.1b, boundaries between the individual and the organisation are overly permeable. From a Gestalt perspective the individual and the organisation are seen to be 'confluent' (Joyce and Sills, 2014) and merged 'as one'. This may be as a result of anxiety about belonging, leading the individual to suppress his or her differences and autonomy for the security of membership. There will be very little differentiation. Conflict will be low, but so will dialogue and learning as there will be little or no exploration of difference and novel perspectives. A coach operating from this position might over-privilege the agenda and norms

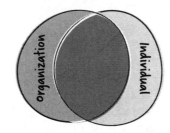

Figure 4.1b Individual and organisation boundaries overly permeable

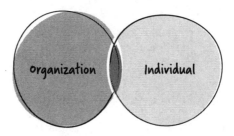

Figure 4.1c Balance between permeability and impermeability

of the organisation and downplay the significance of the coachee's uniqueness and needs.

In Figure 4.1c, there is a balance between sufficient permeability at the contact boundary for the individual to belong and fully contribute to the organisation, while at the same time enough impermeability for the individual to bring his or her autonomy and differences into dialogue with others where this may be optimal. Difference and creative conflict will be tolerated and reflection, inquiry, learning and experimentation are more likely. A coach operating from this perspective is likely to give equal consideration to the requirements of the organisation and the individual needs and perspectives of the coachee. The coach will be interested in how creative dialogue and reciprocal influence might be optimised in service of the mutual beneficial development of individual and organisation.

Given that coaching (and for that matter any intervention that involves people changing how they think and behave as a result) is a personal and private development project occurring in a particular and public context, coaches and coachees have to hold tensions that arise between individual needs, desires and the requirements of the environment. A stance of inquiry and dialogue between the individual and his experience of the environment is more likely to support the creativity and the discovery of new possibilities for both individual coachees and their organisations.

The degree of coachee and coach alignment with the environment, or separateness from it (as set out in the diagrams above), that might represent the most appropriate creative response and resolution of individual needs, role and organisation requirements at any time cannot be pre-determined. Each coach-coachee-context constellation is unique, as are the consequences of particular positions, actions and resolutions in a particular setting at a particular time, and in different contexts within an organisation.

In interacting with peers or superiors a leader may need to assert her difference in the service of innovation, creativity and strategic thinking. In relation to her team, she may need to represent the authority system and forces for compliance and control to a greater extent to ensure necessary management processes and protocols are adhered to.

Personality style, attachment and development histories of coachees and coaches alike can determine whether individuals are more likely to be challenged or seduced by the pull to join with or the pull to separate. The leader in the previous example may be hampered or supported in this on the basis of early experiences and her ability to move fluidly along the continuum from joining with to standing apart. Anxiety in relation to standing apart (and tendency towards merger) might result in her being reluctant to assert herself and her own views with peers and superiors and lead to collusion with reports in order to feel as if she is one of their 'gang'.

In order to be able to adjust to the requirements of the organisation field, collaborate and reconcile at times competing individual, system and operational needs, coaches and coachees need the flexibility to be able to both lean towards alignment with norms, organisation processes and management protocols, or towards differentiation as the situation might require. Conscious and chosen alignment offers a resolution in that the need for individual autonomy, agency and individual choice is protected while also aligning sufficiently with functional contextual norms. Understanding coach and coachee preferences and patterning in either direction opens up the possibility in coaching to develop the capacity for holding the tension of the polarities of joining and separating, thereby facilitating more individual-organisation meeting and dialogue. This can reduce the familiar extremes of unquestioning swallowing of organisational norms as in Figure 4.1b, or reactive rebellious rejection of organisation forces leading to reductionism and limited repertoires as in Figure 4.1a.

More junior employees being coached (and more compliant or anxious coaches for that matter) may feel a stronger pull into merger with the organisation. Equally, the nature of presenting challenges and organisational requirements might indicate that working to strengthen alignment with norms may be optimal. Some senior leaders may feel more permission, may need, or may even have been recruited, to question assumptions and orthodoxies and bring more of their individuality to the organisation (until their difference becomes too much for the context to assimilate, and then they may feel a pull back into alignment with established orthodoxies and patterns). Others still may be inclined to challenge any form of system requirement as in the case of the mavericks who may need to learn to balance their dominant impulse to go against the grain with an increase in capacity to also go along with, as is the case with the 'tempered radical' described by Myerson (2001).

On a larger scale, leaning too far and for too long into alignment with organisational norms risks attrition, rigidity, conformity and totalitarianism (Western, 2012). Here cultural orthodoxies dominate with little or no room for the individual. Whereas, leaning too far in the direction of individual differentiation can lead to chaos, a lack of focus and poor co-ordination of activity. An exploration of the relationship between the coachee and their context, neither privileging one nor the other, enables any paradoxes and tensions to be brought to the surface. This then allows the forces of order and chaos, communion and agency to be negotiated and held more consciously in mind, thereby facilitating conditions in which new meanings and behaviours might emerge. Dimitrov (1997) stresses that the paradoxical and chaotic nature of social reality causes inevitable uncertainty in human decision-making. Where there is uncertainty and vagueness, and where no ultimate answers or obvious best solutions exist, the search for understanding and consensus between people becomes crucial for the management of social complexity. Being able to understand differences in individual thinking and experience provides novelty. Working collaboratively to discover ways to allow this novelty to inform and change existing orthodoxies where necessary is central to organisational change and involves fostering dialogue between the forces for sameness and difference.

From a relational perspective we never can have an individual without an environment, but one pole can come to dominate how the project of coaching and its purpose is constructed by practitioners and their clients. In the context of polarities, privileging the individual over the organisation and vice versa will ultimately lead to the shadow aspects of each position surfacing and interfering with well-being and productivity (Johnson, 1992).

Coaching can offer a space to affirm and confirm each coachee's uniqueness and desire, allowing each to have and express a mind of his own. At the same time, it needs to offer the opportunity to explore the necessary compromises and negotiation of differences between individual and context, person and role. In this way coachees can experience support and recognition for what is important to them and who they know themselves to be, while also adopting roles that are both meaningful to them and appropriate to the task and context. They can explore the compromises they are prepared to make, and also whether there is anything about their role or context that they find fundamentally compromises their sense of integrity. Where clients feel fundamentally and intolerably compromised, they may need also to explore whether they can continue in good faith in the organisation. Helping clients to differentiate between unconscious reactivity based on the past, and adult aware choice based on the present moment situation is vital here.

Adopting a role with relevant skills and taking on a work identity means shaping a part of the self in a specific direction. Levine (2010) stresses that, while it is important not only that an individual be able to do so, it is equally crucial that 'the individual not disappear altogether into his or her work role because our professional identity leaves aside much of what is vital about us' (p. 119). This capacity for vitality is central to enlivening organisations and unlocking innovation and creative potential.

Difficult differences – The 'maverick'

Over the years we have worked with individuals who are described as mavericks in their organisations. Often this means that they possess a number of qualities that are seen as desirable by the organisation and frequently they are extremely successful in terms of getting results, but something about their way of doing business or interacting with others clashes with cultural and organisational norms. More often than not it is their willingness to be different that is central to their success, and yet it is also this very difference that can create a tension at the boundary between them as individuals and the norms of the wider organisation. Different organisational cultures tolerate, welcome and make use of difference to varying degrees. Culture, the seniority of the individual, risk and the perceived ratio of 'gain' to 'risk' all have a bearing on this. Different coachees with maverick tendencies will have varying degrees of capacity and willingness to compromise some of their difference where this is creating difficulties for them in relation to the context they find themselves in. We have found it useful to explore themes of sameness and difference with coachees, always from a perspective of the coachee being the only one who can decide ultimately the degree of alignment with or difference from norms, as it is she who has to live with the consequences of her choices. Membership in human systems and organisations always requires some degree of compromise of individual preferences. This can be a revelation to those who may be in the grip of an old relational template where any form of compromise or requirement from the environment is experienced as an impinging demand or as suffocating of their individuality. Coachees can be helped to explore these tensions and choose the degree of compromise that they can bear in order to function in the organisation. They then have the opportunity to deploy their talents in ways that the organisation can value and make use of, rather than their difference primarily eliciting anxiety, concern and an impulse to control them in the wider system. This can create conditions where differences can be explored in order to discover what they might have to offer both the coachee and context.

Forces for sameness – The organisational context

While all organisations need norms and structures to confer stability and appropriate degrees of control, where these become overly dominant they can stifle creativity and innovation, suppressing individuality, dulling the human spirit and leading to a cult-like system of conformity. It is interesting for us to note that a common feature of totalitarian societies is legislation that prevents individuals from meeting in groups for conversation that is not contained or stage-managed by the authorities (Arieli and Rotenstreich, 2002). These 'authorities' know all too well that when people come together, meet and converse, real change risks actually happening!

We might conclude that living in a democracy is fundamentally different to such a context. While it may be true that many of us do not live in systems that so overtly attempt to police thought, there is much that can be applied from an understanding of these processes and their psychological underpinnings that can be relevant to a relational orientation to coaching.

Organisations implicitly and explicitly establish expectations about what is required of their members to fit in, activating anxiety in members in relation to differences and, where more primitive survival needs are fused with work success and financial reward, fear of exclusion and ejection for some.

Schwartz (1990) writing from within the psychoanalytic tradition has demonstrated how the self-image and aspirational identity of individuals or 'ego ideal' becomes fused with the ideals of the organisation and brand image. As such it becomes extremely difficult to raise any issue or perspective that might challenge the individual and organisational ideals. The nature of belonging here is essentially narcissistic with individual identity being inseparable from the image that the organisation and its members want to project. There is no room for a wider range of subjectivity. Data or phenomena that in some way threaten the organisational ideal are ignored or disappeared, as seen in numerous examples of whistleblowing or corporate failure. Here illegal and dangerous practices are eventually exposed, often due to some catastrophic consequence of inappropriate actions and choices, which have been hidden for years in order to maintain in the minds of employees and the general public, the organisation's image of viability, integrity and success.

Strong brand identity and loyalty can and do also give rise to contexts that support creativity and innovation. In the post modern era, Western (2012) argues that the identity and belonging that organisations offer is necessary for containing anxiety given the lack of grand narratives that individuals might have identified with in the past such as religion or nationalism. By the same token, this can also lead to individuals feeling 'dislocated and worn down. Global corporations, corporate hotels, international airports and global shopping malls merge into a bland, minimalist oneness, dulling our spirits' (p. 108). What are sacrificed, given the pursuit of what Garvey *et al.* (2009) term the 'benefits of control' are the 'energizing advantages of liberation and personal responsibility' (p. 160.). As is the case with narcissism we risk becoming brittle, limited, homogenous and empty facsimiles, disconnected from the vitalising quality of diversity and fuller uniquely embodied subjectivity. Employees become 'split subjects – they feel whole, aligned and engaged as part of the brand community, yet at the same time feel lost, empty inside and dislocated' (Deleuze and Guattari, 2004, pp. 7–8, cited in Western, 2012, p. 111).

The pressure to 'fit in' and identify with organisation ideals can make it difficult for some coachees to experience or express any feeling or thought that is considered to be unacceptable in relation to the prevailing organisational ideology. Organisations can tightly prescribe the parameters of coaching and what is and is not acceptable to explore. These boundaries can infiltrate the coaching relationship leading to anxiety between coaches and coachees about what is permissible and, if unexamined, can narrow the space for potential discovery (Cavicchia and Fillery Travis, 2013). Given the privileging of the rational in most organisations, any expression of feeling other than passionate optimism and loyalty to the organisation and its ideals may be off limits, at least publicly! Some common understanding of organisational expectations and norms is important for defining the organisation. Yet these beliefs and structures can also become, as has been identified in the psychoanalytic literature on organisational life, rigid, institutional defences against anxiety which, if not acknowledged, limit the range and adaptability of individuals and the organisation in the face of constant change in both external and internal environments (Armstrong, 2005; Czander, 1993; Gould *et al.*, 2001; Hirschhorn and Barnett, 1993; Obholzer and Zagier-Roberts, 1994; Vansina and Vansina-Cobbaert, 2008).

From a relational, contextual and intersubjective perspective we are interested in researching with our clients their direct experience, the field conditions in which they operate and the interplay between the two. This is particularly necessary in the VUCA environment given the need to make sufficient sense of complexity, experiment with new behaviours and strategic possibilities, and where work and the knowledge economy demand 'the cognitive, creative and subjective self be active ingredients of labour' (Western, 2012, p. 259).

This is where coaching can support coachees, particularly in executive coaching, to understand and make use of emotions and understanding of their self-organising process to also meet company requirements, all the while holding the tension of the individual and the context in dialogue. This can reduce the negative consequences of leaning too far toward either end of the individual-organisation continuum – as Western (2012) states, 'working towards efficiency and company success is vital, but not if it undermines morale, or creates blind spots with serious human consequences' (p. 187).

Over the years we have found ourselves coming up against boundaries and fixed ideas in the minds of clients around what is acceptable within their context.

Coaching and change – The challenging potential of novelty

Many learning and human development traditions such as Gestalt (Gaffney, 2010, 2011; Nevis, 1987), action learning (Pedler, 2012) and approaches based on constructivist developmental psychology (Fisher *et al.*, 2003) acknowledge that for growth and learning to occur, individuals must experience an encounter with novelty, expanding perceptual frames and experimenting with new strategies that are different to familiar patterns of thought and action in individuals and the organisations they shape.

Against the backdrop of the aspects of organisational life we have outlined, it can be difficult as a coach to hold the degree of marginality necessary to be sufficiently novel or 'other' to support and challenge clients to experience and perceive things differently, in a way that is beneficial to their development and their organisation's success. Barber (2006b) suggests this phenomenon is, in part, due to the way 'organisations make collective demands on the individual that infiltrate and subjugate them to a collective consciousness which sucks them into the personality structure of the group' (p. 78).

There can be an enormous pressure for coachees and coaches alike to align with the usual and familiar ways organisations and their members construct their versions of reality. This will not always be problematic. There may be occasions when clients and coaches choose to be more aligned with the demands of the organisation, where this is seen to be the most effective way of supporting the interests of both the individual and the enterprise. An example of this would be development coaching where coaching is overtly positioned to support individuals to develop skills, behaviours and working practices aligned with an organisation's strategy. At other times, attending to the needs of the business might call for experimentation with different perspectives, as in the case of executive coaching and transformational learning where new perspectives, new knowledge and action may be called for in the face of complex and challenging environments. Traditional assumptions about positional power and hierarchy may need to be deconstructed in line with post modern and complexity perspectives that suggest that power and influence reside potentially in all members of an organisation and move between different members at different times (Laloux, 2014).

In this way it can be seen that the relationship of individual to environment has a dialectic quality to it, at times leaning into alignment with norms, at other times calling forth more individual creativity and challenge.

Challenges for the coach's 'self-organisation'

Faced with an individual or organisation strongly wedded (often unconsciously) to a particular dominant set of assumptions about behaviour and what may be required to be a good corporate citizen, it can feel difficult for coaches to inquire and raise awareness in a way that calls into question some of the assumptions which underpin it. In working to develop a more intersubjective feedback culture in an information technology organisation (Coffey and Cavicchia, 2005), I (SC) and my colleague discovered that the organisation's ideals of perfection were actually contributing to making it difficult for people to develop, as there was little room for making mistakes in order to learn. Falling short of an ideal of perfection was experienced by individuals as deeply shaming. As a result, a culture of politeness and platitudes had developed where difficult performance conversations and developmental feedback were avoided.

A working assumption underpinning a relational orientation to coaching is that coaches be willing to use their own differences and subjectivity to act as a catalytic force for change, offering an experience to the client of an 'other' with whom the client can explore new possibilities. This could sound challenging to notions of the coach being some kind of neutral force whose job it is to play down his or her differences, knowledge and perspectives in order to draw out the latent and innate knowing of his client.

From a relational and intersubjective perspective, the idea of pure neutrality is problematic. All coaches will have their biases, prior knowledge, training backgrounds. These inevitably, in subtle and not so subtle ways, influence what the coach feels and thinks in relation to her coachee and how she makes meaning. What remains crucial is that the coach can make her differences available in the form of thoughts, perspectives, reactions and responses to the coachee. In this way the coach uses her 'otherness', offers it for the coachee to engage with in order to discover his own versions of meaning that have resonance and relevance for him and his context. The coach endeavours to remain unattached to any specific outcome, attachment to which would increase the likelihood of pressure being applied to the coachee to comply with what the coach believes to be right. We shall explore this practice orientation further in Section 2.

Daring to make use of our differences and marginality in the context of coaching and fully making our subjective otherness available to the conversation is not without its challenges. Yet as Critchley (2012) stresses this is fundamental to a relational orientation to coaching rooted in social constructionist and inter-subjective ideas that client and coach are engaged in a process of reciprocal influence, creating one another by shaping each other's experience, where meaning arises in the process of relating. The coach in this orientation does not 'do to' or 'act upon' the client, nor does he act as an instrument in service of the client but as an 'other' with whom the client can interact. As Critchley (2012) states, if a coach attempts to withhold him or herself in the interests of impartiality or detachment, this will reduce the creative possibility inherent in a process of fully relating.

This way of working can feel very different for coach and coachee alike to the more instrumental and dry processes that underpin much traditional performance related coaching. These serve to keep both parties relatively safe and protected from the risk of fully embodied relating, preferring to align with protocols and coaching orthodoxies, rather than opening to the direct experience of being in relation and what this might allow in terms of difference, learning and development.

Our own experience, and that of students and supervisees, have taught us that coaches can feel anxious when it comes to naming directly aspects of our coachees's relating that have impacted us. We might feel exposed, when exploring our coachee's context, in raising awareness of ways in which an organisation falls short of living up to its own ideals, or when naming what Schein (1988) terms 'disconfirming data'. This is where the actual experience and behaviour of individuals, or 'theory in use', does not align with the 'espoused theory' (Argyris, 1999). The very act of seeing things differently, or 'looking awry' (Western, 2012) can, at times, feel subversive and the coach might be seen as adopting the role of the child in the fairy tale of the emperor's new clothes.

Where attachment to norms, ideals and fixed ideas is particularly strong in an organisation, as coaches we can experience a complete incapacity to think and make connections in our minds. We can feel as if we are being induced into merging with the organisation's version of reality as embodied by our coaching client. We might find ourselves unable to access any curiosity and love of inquiry, which we may have come to trust and rely upon as practitioners. When this happens, it can often be a sign of our clients' own difficulties with thinking beyond their system's 'propaganda' and their internalisation of it. From a relational perspective, it is clear that, at times like this, difference and, therefore, change and growth will inevitably be diminished. 'Thinking outside the box' has now become a cliché in organisational consulting, yet it remains exceedingly difficult in these organisations to do, especially when attachment to maintaining the familiarity of the box can be so great.

Even where there is more need and support for questioning in the system, we can often feel exposed if our comments and associations set us apart as 'other' to the system. We can encounter our own anxieties about belonging and concerns regarding securing work by giving clients a degree of what they 'want' as opposed to what may be 'required' for development and context-relevant change to occur. Depending on our personality and attachment styles we might even feel as if our viability and survival as practitioners is under threat.

This can be at once grounded in reality, in that a client could resort to rejecting our perspectives and eject us from the system, *and* also be a resonance with our clients' anxiety at the prospect of facing a more complex perspective on their organisation and their role within it than they had previously considered. This, in turn, might result in them feeling set apart from the mainstream. Shaw and Stacey (2006) suggest that anxiety is a necessary and inevitable part of all change processes. Reflection and inquiry can often lead to implications and consequences that clients may be reluctant to acknowledge and be unsupported (initially) to act upon. This is not to say that they always *need* to be acted upon, but rather, allowed to surface in order that they might be considered for what they have to offer and support more creativity and aware response ability.

In being sufficiently 'other' to allow for dialogue and change, we can feel to some extent that we are risking. Risking that our difference will be too alien for a client to engage with, risking that our willingness to be vulnerable and sit with 'not knowing' will be interpreted through a 'performance excellence' bias as incompetence and result in reputational damage. These feelings often mirror the experience of coachees who might also be experimenting with allowing more feelings and a broader range of thinking into their repertoire in contexts that may be wedded to particular perspectives and norms. Acknowledging the mutual risk coach and coachee might encounter can go a long way towards normalising the experience of exposure. Also, as working alliances develop and deepen, and the coachee has experiences of the catalytic, permission giving, expansive and energising potential that emerges in fuller human to human contact (without necessarily even having to do or aim for anything), both coach and coachee can begin to trust more in the process of relating and exploring differences for what they might offer. Then being occasionally too different, wild or 'wacky' stands more of a chance of being accepted and explored. It raises the need to consider what support (for both) might be needed to ensure safe emergency of new perspectives and practice.

A relational approach to coaching requires that the coach also be willing to bring more of him/herself to the meeting with clients, including those aspects that may have little support in the organisational field. Managing and making use of a wider range of feelings and thoughts, finding internal and external support in the form of appropriate supervision and membership of sufficiently like-minded communities of practice, which also welcome and can contain diversity, represent core competences for any coach interested in incorporating more of a relational orientation into their work. In this way our own expanded range can support our clients to access more of themselves in service of their development and effectiveness.

This means that at times the process of relating between coach and coachee is likely to be messy, as each attempts to understand the other and each negotiates the implications of differences between them. This represents another departure from a view of coaching, which is highly structured, with specific tools and exercises used in a particular order, and where the coach might presume to know broadly what outcomes might be. With the right conditions, which we shall explore in more detail in the next section, coachees and coaches can learn to negotiate continuity and change (Bromberg, 1996), exploring what is familiar and also what novel possibilities there might be for growth and development to occur. In this way coaching can become a space in which to play as described by the psychoanalyst Donald Winnicott (1996). A place in which room can be made for the minds of coach and coachee to wander and allow anything that arises to be considered for its possible relevance to the client and their development, rather than tightly policing in advance what might be considered appropriate to talk about.

Example

At the first session with a senior executive in a multi-national organisation, the coach made time to remind the client of the way he works. He explained that he sees his job as reflecting with clients on the nature of their organisational challenges and how they perceive them, with a view to both coach and coachee working to discover what might support resolution of challenges within the coachee and the wider organisation.

The coach was curious, therefore, during the next few meetings, about the frequency with which the coachee would ask (often in a rather sheepish way that contrasted with the confidence he displayed when talking about his work) whether the coach thought the session was going well.

The coach felt a pull into giving his assessment of the work so far. After all, this was a very senior client, making a direct request. Surely he must respond to it? He started to scan his recollection of the work to date, the conceptual frameworks he was drawing upon, and prepared to launch into a fulsome (and undoubtedly polished!) commentary. Yet, just as he was about to speak, he became aware of a nagging concern. Something did not feel right. He felt as if he were being invited to do all the work, and pass judgement in a rather one-sided, authoritative way. He found himself imagining soothing and reassuring the client, and became curious about what this might be revealing about him, the coachee and the relationship. He reined himself in and commented:

'On a number of occasions now you have asked me for my assessment of our work together and I find myself curious about what might be happening for you when you do this.'

The response he received was immediate and tinged with a considerable amount of anger.

'Well you're the coach, you should know where it needs to be going!'

The coach was taken aback by the force of the coachee's response. He felt himself slipping into some familiar shaming self-talk about how he was getting it wrong by not meeting his client's overt expectations, and how he was risking his reputation with a client who was important to him (and his portfolio!).

He supported himself by returning in his mind to part of the original contract he had agreed with the client to create space for reflection, and reminded the coachee of how, if he were willing, it might be worth pausing for a moment to pay attention to what was happening between them. The coachee seemed slightly taken aback by this response before breaking into a curious, inviting smile.

The coach wondered aloud what the coachee's looking to him to determine whether the session was going well might be saying about the organisation and his relationship to it.

This seemed to open the floodgates. The coachee became visibly animated and spoke about how his organisation had very clear guidelines for how to think, speak and behave, and that senior managers were expected to be the gatekeepers for these behaviours, communicating them and policing them.

He quickly saw for himself that he had brought this dynamic into the room and projected the role of 'judge' of what constituted success on to the coach, seeing him as an embodiment of the organisation's orthodoxies and authority given that his services had been procured by the organisation.

This allowed the coach to restate that, as far as he was concerned, there were two people in the room, each with the capacity to determine how well the work might was going. The coach, on the basis of his background and understanding of coaching, organisations and human relating. The coachee, on the basis of the extent to which he experienced being able to use what emerged in the sessions to support himself to work more effectively in his context. The coach also suggested that, at times, they may not agree. Far from implying this was problematic, he speculated that this might actually provide fruitful contact and dialogue where their differences might prove to be the source of new perspectives . . . for both of them!

This seemed to shift something. The coach experienced himself relaxing and becoming more present, allowing thoughts and associations to arise without a need to pin them down in the form of an assessment. The coachee too seemed to connect more deeply with his own experience and thoughts, holding them lightly and relishing the space, as he put it to 'play with possibilities'.

Over time, the coachee came increasingly to value the coaching space (physical, temporal and psychological), make use of it to think more freely, and consider what he might do differently outside of the meetings. He would still experience anxiety at having thoughts that differed from the organisational ideal of unquestioning compliance. The coach was openly able to link this to his own anxiety when the client initially asked him for his assessment of the session and both saw how each could experience self-doubt and shame when their experience and thinking seemed to run counter to the environment's expectations (the client's request for the coach's opinion which was not expected by the coach, the client's experience and thinking in relation to the organisation). Coach and coachee would then spend time considering what interventions the coachee might make, and how they might be graded so that his colleagues might at least consider what he had to say.

The sessions enabled the coachee to find the support to question and challenge received ways of thinking and doing that had outgrown their effectiveness and were actually hampering efficiency in the wider field, and in his department in particular.

This vignette serves to illustrate how clients can project aspects of the context and culture onto the coach, particularly the organisation's preoccupation with expertise. The coachee was later able to talk about his frustration with the coach when he resisted giving him his assessment of the coaching, which, at one level, the coachee thought he wanted so much. They surfaced together that the coachee needed to believe that the coach knew what he was doing (signified, interestingly, by expert opinion rather than process, facilitation and inquiry expertise) given his own, more private, levels of anxiety. By both of them finding the support to stay with an inquiry-mindedness in relation to what was happening between them, the coachee was able to connect more with his own mental and creative resources and reclaim the capability he was initially so willing to project onto the coach.

At times this brought the coachee into conflict with his line manager who was still operating on the basis of unquestioned assumptions about power and deference to hierarchy. The coachee used his coaching to explore how to build a stronger relationship with his manager and experiment with a range of ways of introducing his own new perspectives. Over time, while this was not always easy, he reported a better working relationship and greater dialogue with his superior, resulting in modifications to some existing processes which both he and his manager could agree needed attention. While there are no guarantees that working in this way will always yield a successful outcome for the coachee and organisation, we hope it serves to illustrate that the consequences of questioning the ways in which orthodoxies shape experience and experimentation with different strategies need not be quite as catastrophic as can be imagined by coaches and coachees experiencing the pressure to comply with dominant and familiar cultural patterns and behavioural expectations.

Section 2

Practice perspectives

Chapter 5

Coming together
Unpacking the coach-coachee-context constellation

When we extend the framing of coaching beyond primarily the application of models and tools for facilitating one to one learning, and take a wider perspective on human intersubjectivity and the importance of context in shaping individual experience, meaning making and possibilities for action, it is possible to begin to consider a host of factors that subtly and not so subtly come together to inform the coach-coachee-context constellation.

These are the forces and factors in the coach, the coachee and context that make every meeting and engagement a unique universe. They stand to shape the individual experience of coach and coachee, the coaching relationship, the conversation that unfolds, the work that is done, the meaning that is made and the outcomes that might be achieved.

Quantum perspectives (Bohm, 2002; Mindell, 2000; Wheatley, 2001) suggest that how we look determines in large part what we see. The personalities, biases and backgrounds of coach and coachee, including training, theoretical and ethical orientation, will all contribute to how we perceive and how we make sense of any situation in particular ways. These inevitably result in illuminating and emphasising certain aspects of a situation, while also disappearing or missing others that might be potentially relevant for learning and development to occur. From the perspective of theoretical integration, being able to shift perceptual frames and theoretical lenses can increase the range of ways in which we and our clients might tentatively make meaning from any experience. This then stands to increase the range of choices that can emerge to experiment with different perspectives and working assumptions, along with the behaviours they give rise to. This is supported by neuroscience perspectives (Azmatullah, 2013; Siegel, 2010), which stress the importance for health and the development of increasing range of perception, experience and meaning making beyond fixed and recurring patterns of thinking and acting.

When coach and coachee come together as two subjectivities in interaction, they stand to influence one another as well as be influenced by the context in which the work is happening. The discovery of mirror neurons (di Pellegrino *et al.*, 1992; Gallese, 2001; Gallese and Goldman, 1998) further supports understanding of the powerful ways in which humans influence and shape one another's experience. Mirror neurons are neurons that fire in the brains of individuals observing an other perform a particular action, for example picking up an object. Their name derives from the fact that they are the same neurons that fire when the observer actually performs the task that has been observed. They are also seen to be connected to the learning of manual skills, the evolution of gestural communication, spoken language, group cohesion and empathy (Cozolino, 2006). Mirror neurons are implicated in the experience of resonance, how we find ourselves connecting with and resonating with the experience of an other. It is this capacity for resonance that enables coaches and coachees to understand one another and make explicit meaning together from the more implicit felt experience of being together which has not yet been articulated in language. Coaches can make use of the felt experience of being with their clients to formulate interventions which are attuned to their client's experience in the moment and can heighten the client's awareness of how they are constructing themselves and their reality. We shall expand on this in the following chapters. Mirror neurons also shed light on why coachees can, and often do, change simply from being in the presence of a coach who models a calm, attuned, responsive, reflective and relational attitude.

Intersubjective (Orange, 1994), Gestalt (Wheeler, 2000) relational psychoanalytic (Aron, 1996; 1999) and neuroscience (Schore, 2003) perspectives all point to the transformative potential of conversation and relationship. Cavanagh (2006), drawing primarily on the work of Stacey (2001), has suggested that coaching can be thought about as a complex adaptive conversation. Here, knowing, meaning and change are seen as properties emerging from the interaction and dynamics between coach and coachee. Both are inevitably shaped by their individual histories and life contexts and stand to influence and shape one another in a process of reciprocal influence in the coaching conversation.

For Jung the relationship dynamics between practitioner and client are seen as the crucible or alchemical bath in which both stand to be changed (Jacoby, 1984; Samuels, 1985). Thomas Ogden (1994) describes a view of relationship where a 'third' space opens up between the two individuals participating in the conversation. In this spatial metaphor individual subjectivities meet and influence one another at conscious and unconscious, explicit and implicit levels. Associations, images and thoughts arise in the crucible of this meeting. These perspectives on the interactive and mutually influencing properties of relationships explain how it is that with some clients we might find ourselves feeling settled, calm and where the conversation seems to flow, thoughts, associations, insights, responses and strategies come readily to mind, and there is a feeling of effortlessness, fluidity and ease. Whereas, with others, we might feel heavy, anxious, blank, unsure how to proceed, and the conversation seems laboured. Opening and attuning to the subtle ways in which coach and client experience themselves and influence one another can unlock much potential discovery and meaning making for coachees and coaches alike.

We shall describe in detail ways in which coaches might work with this orientation in Chapter 8.

These ideas stand in marked contrast to approaches based primarily on individualist assumptions of doer and done to, linear approaches to change, over-reliance on tools and stage models, and communication seen as a process of transmission. Instead communication is seen as a series of gestures and responses (Mead and Morris, 1967; Stacey, 2000). One party will speak or act, the content (explicit dimension) and the manner and feeling tone (implicit dimension) of which have an impact on the other based on their resonance, meaning making and subjective uniqueness. This in turn is what generates their next response, which impacts the other and so on. While the impacts of some gestures might be predictable to some extent, for example being critical of someone might result in a counter attack or a hurt pulling away from relationship, it is never possible to know exactly the precise contours and subtleties of how these processes will unfold. The sociologist George Herbert Mead succinctly describes this process when he says that the 'meaning of a gesture by one organism is found in the response of the other organism' (Mead and Morris, 1967, p. 147 cited in Critchley, 2010). We might have a particular intention in relation to an other, but the meaning of the gesture reveals itself in the other's response. A coach, informed by coaching protocol, may suggest to a coachee that he email the coach when he has completed an action related to the client's development objectives. The coach's intention may be to support the client to achieve his goals and bring focus and accountability to the coachee and the coaching process, an intervention seen as a core competence in the accreditation of coaches by some accrediting bodies. It cannot be known until the coachee responds (or not!), and in what manner, whether the coach's gesture is construed and experienced by this particular coachee as helpful, or as irritating, invasive and infantilising. Paying close attention to the dynamics of gesture and response is a central component of a relational orientation to coaching as it is the territory where patterns of thought and action reveal themselves and meanings emerge for consideration and re-evaluation where necessary.

This is yet another challenge to the deterministic assumption that can still persist in some practitioners and coachees that there is the 'right' intervention to make that will have a predictable, powerful and beneficial impact. Much energy is often expended, and self-doubt activated, in trying to get it 'right', as if this can be known in advance. From a relational perspective all interventions on the part of the coach can be seen as 'informed gestures', the impact of which cannot be fully known, or sometimes even known at all in advance. A key component to the coaching relationship is to discover together with the coachee what uses she is able, and chooses, to put the coach and the relationship to in service of her learning and the requirements of context. These uses can be overt and explicit as well as less visible but nonetheless significant. Viewed from this perspective, coaching is less about primarily driving for pre-determined and specified results, but needs also to include sensitivity and close attention to creating conditions and practices which might support less predictable and potentially even more generative conversations to happen (see Chapter 8). This can go some way to liberating coaches from the tyranny of perfectionism, but is certainly not a licence to be uncensored or unthinking in how we interact with another human being. What coaches find themselves saying and how they participate in the co-creation of meaning and coaching outcomes with their coachees will be informed by a host of factors, including their experience, knowledge and blind spots, as well as the particular dynamics of the coach-coachee-context constellation.

One way, therefore, to think of relational coaching and collaborative meaning making is as a form of 'bricolage'. In French, 'bricolage' is used to mean 'tinkering' (in the craft sense, not interfering!) or 'pottering', in the service of creating something from a diverse range of inputs. The term 'social bricolage' was coined by the cultural anthropologist Claude Levi-Strauss (1968) who was interested in the ways in which societies create novel solutions by using resources, including ways of thinking and acting, that already exist in the social consciousness. Social psychologists, drawing on the work of Lévi-Strauss (1968) as well as the process of 'creative cognition', an intra-psychic approach to studying the ways in which people retrieve and recombine knowledge in new ways (Finke, 1996), use theterm 'psychological bricolage'. This refers to the mental processes that are involved in individuals creating new solutions by using hitherto unrelated knowledge or ideas they already possess (Sanchez-Burks, Karlesky and Lee, 2015). Sanchez-Burks *et al*. (2015) go on to demonstrate how different skills and strategies are associated with different versions of self we might experience in different contexts. Coaching can support coachees to access skills and capacities associated with identities they may have or have had outside of the workplace and enable them to transfer these, where appropriate, into their professional lives.

A coaching client had recently been promoted to a more senior leadership role which required him to develop greater systemic understanding and the ability to perceive patterns and signals in his organisation in order to monitor how individuals were responding to a series of major strategic changes. Initially he found this a very daunting prospect given that his prior management training was steeped in linear and logical assumptions of command and control. He was not used to accessing his sensations and intuition, and was missing opportunities for intervening early to make necessary course corrections on the basis of more subtle and weak signals from the environment. As his coach supported him to orient to what cultivating system sensitivity might look and feel like, the coachee suddenly remembered a time many years earlier when he was working as a nightclub bouncer. This association evoked in him memories of being able to intuit early when a situation might be about to get out of hand or turn violent. His coach invited him to track his experience of the memory and see if he could sense into and describe this past experience in more detail in the present moment. The coachee remembered that he would initially become alert to a slight change in the pattern of behaviour among a throng of people on the dancefloor. This would be accompanied by a 'gut feel' of apprehension followed by alertness and greater focus on the specific area that had captured his attention. This memory was a powerful catalyst in enabling the coachee to connect with more intuitive and somatic intelligence to complement his reason and logic, and supported him to achieve his development objectives.

Relevant to the practice of 'bricolage' Stacey (2000) has identified the importance of connectivity and diversity in creating conversations that are generative and developmental. Connectivity refers to the richness of themes and associations within the conversation. Diversity refers to supplying novelty, difference and tension from a wide range of fields and sources. This provides important levels of misunderstanding (which can be explored for its meaning) and cross-fertilisation needed to stimulate novel connections. We shall explore some of the processes involved here and how they may be made use of in coaching in the following chapters.

We want now to set out some of the different factors, fields and sources that inform interactions and give rise to coaching intervention gestures and 'bricolage' in the relational system that is the coach-coachee-context constellation. The Gestalt writer Malcolm Parlett (2015) describes 'that people are basically different all the time, and vary according to the total situation which they are currently experiencing – as well as, in part, constructing' (pp. 66–67).

The following perspectives offer a window onto different factors that might, to varying degrees, be contributing to the 'total situation' coach and coachee find themselves in at any particular point in time. This is not intended to be an exhaustive list, but an invitation to coaches to consider some of the ways in which their own and their coachees' thinking and practice *may* be being shaped and the form it might take in different contexts, as well as new forms it might take by considering the bringing together of different elements, accessing what Western (2012) terms 'associative intelligence'.

In this way coaches might become increasingly aware of, and able to reflect on these processes, the particular attachments they might have to certain ways of seeing things, and expand their range for thinking and acting. This lies at the heart of both relational coaching and supervisory processes. To the extent that the person we are is the coach that we are, the more awareness, range and flexibility we can find in ourselves and our own meaning making patterns, stands to increase the range and space we can offer to our coachees to explore, where appropriate, the intricacies of their experience in their contexts. What constitutes an effective intervention is a function of multiple factors including coach personality, skill, sensitivity, reflexivity, attunement to self and other, pre-existing knowledge, as well as that generated together, along with the coachee's capacity to make use of it in their context. We hope thinking in this way might support coaches and our coachees to be open to seeing meaning and meaning making as a socially co-emergent process. This stands to facilitate greater exploration and understanding of different perceptual frames, and relax rigid pre-reflective over identification (Welwood, 2000) and attachments to one protocol, one way of thinking, or having to be 'right' based on tried and tested methodologies presumed to be generalisable in all situations. This allows for meanings to be held more lightly, and existing thinking and assumptions to relax, in order for new perspectives and possibilities to emerge and be experimented with, as is the case with reflective practice, action learning and transformational approaches to coaching (Cox, 2013; Fisher, Torbert and Rooke, 2000; Mezirow, 1990; Oliver, 2010).

Sentient essence – From where does meaning come?

Quantum mechanics is a branch of physics concerned with the properties and behaviour of sub atomic particles considered to be the building blocks of matter. It has postulated that what we see at this micro level seems to be directly affected by what we look for, which has implications for the way in which perceptions of reality and meaning are constructed (Khrennikov, 2014). Increasingly, these and other discoveries are having wide reaching implications in fields such as philosophy, psychology and the study of consciousness. The work of physicist, Jungian analyst and founder of process psychology Arnold Mindell (2000) points to the relationship between quantum physics, consciousness and reality. He proposes a model of reality made up of three domains – consensus reality, dreaming and sentient essence. Consensus reality consists of the differing perceptions of individuals that correspond with one another. This is the realm of forms such as tables and chairs, ideas, beliefs and theories, which appear as separate and distinct. Yet at the quantum, sub atomic level, all matter – the desks we sit at at work, our living bodies, thought forms and mental constructions – is made up of energy in the form of particles and waves. For some, these quantum perspectives point to a deeper unity or 'oneness' behind the surface appearance of things which resonates with ideas, beliefs and orientations to reality from a number of spiritual traditions, especially those of the East. The physicist David Bohm (2002) dedicated much of his life to exploring and understanding the nature of, and processes involved in, human dialogue. For many years he was in conversation with the spiritual teacher Jiddu Krishnamurthi (1985) and his work has greatly influenced the dialogue work of William Isaacs (1999). What all these thinkers have in common is a deep commitment to understanding human relating through the medium of dialogue and exploring how it can be used to bring people together, inquire and create new meanings and possibilities.

Mindell suggests that it is extremely difficult for change to happen at the level of consensus reality (2000). This is partly because we become attached to the meanings, forms and mental constructs which we can then take to be *the* truth, defending them, selecting data to reinforce them and closing to other data, experiences and phenomena which might call their rigidity and absoluteness into question. In order for changes in meaning to occur we need to orient our consciousness to what Mindell terms the 'dreaming'. This is the realm of consciousness where attachment to positions and familiar perceptual frames relaxes and new possibilities for experience, thinking and acting might emerge. It is the realm of feeling and direct experience, intuition, the imaginal (Heron, 1999), and is the realm we invite our clients into when we ask them to drop into sensing their bodies, follow their sensory experience, work with imagery or metaphor, sense deeply into feeling what captures their attention internally and externally and what matters to them. Mindell (2001; 2002), Isaacs (1999) and change thinkers such as Scharmer (2009) have developed a series of practices which can be used to facilitate accessing the 'dreaming', letting go of attachment to familiar beliefs and letting new possibilities and perspectives come in the service of new learning and transformational action (Scharmer and Kaufer, 2013). Beneath the 'dreaming' Mindell describes the quantum field of particles and waves as 'sentient essence'. As is the case in many spiritual traditions, he considers this 'essence' to be consciousness itself – the formless undifferentiated ground from which all forms, including meaning, emerge.

While these ideas and perspectives might seem complex and esoteric to some, many of them are already informing coaching theory such as ontological perspectives which pay attention to the experience of being and study how the ways in which we construct reality is fundamental to how we formulate problems, shape our limitations and unlock potential (Olalla, 2010); presence focused coaching (Silsbee, 2008) and integral coaching (Flaherty, 2010), as well as complexity theory and dialogue practices being applied in organisations. What they offer is an opportunity to broaden perspective beyond consensus realities, relax attachments to particular schools or approaches, explore how meaning emerges in human relations, look 'awry' (Western, 2012) and question those meanings that may have become overly fixed, unhelpfully limiting or harmful in some way. They support the process of transformational learning whereby new meanings and choices for action beyond pre-existing paradigms can be generated. When we become more sensitised to our embodied felt sense of being in the present moment, and the ways in which we might be constructing our reality on the basis of our particular assumptions and patterns of thought, we can be open to apprehending the qualities of the wider fields and contexts which subtly influence how we experience ourselves, others and make meaning together. This supports greater critical reflection on the situations we find ourselves in and how we make sense of them which, in turn, supports greater range of choice and experimentation with new possibilities.

Drawing on ideas from existentialism and social constructionism, Thompson (2016) emphasises that human experience is best understood in terms of three interconnecting levels: the personal, cultural and structural. These levels recognise that individuals (Personal level) do not operate in a vacuum and are strongly influenced by meaning frameworks which shape their perception of the world (the Cultural level). The cultural level in turn does not operate in a vacuum, but is located within a wide context of social structures (the Structural level). This points to the fact that society is not neutral or a level playing field, but operates according to a series of social divisions such as class, race/ethnicity, gender etc. It is a limitation of the individualistic orientation that it focuses only on the personal level and discounts the wider cultural and structural dimensions that inevitably influence human experience, meaning making and action. Thompson (2016) references a metaphor attributed to Sartre (1956), which demonstrates how individual self-experience and the wider field are enmeshed. Traditional approaches to human psychology have tended to view the individual as central and the social context as a passive background to human action, rather like soup in a bowl. Here the soup represents the individual who is contained and constrained by the bowl but where there is a clear impermeable boundary between soup and bowl so that each remains a distinct and separate entity (Elkjaer, 2005 cited in Thompson, 2016). For Sartre (1956) human experience in context is more akin to coffee and cream where, once mixed together, they become a new entity, rather than two entities side by side.

From an existentialist perspective, this metaphor captures more accurately the complexities of human existence in which aspects of our wider social and organisational contexts become part of us and us part of the wider social situation. This has significant implications for a relational and contextual view of coaching and the coach-coachee-context constellation. From this perspective coach and coachee are shaped and moulded by context while also standing to influence context and one another. The coffee and cream metaphor points to how a new entity comes into being when coffee mixes with cream. This is not to say that coffee and cream cease to exist, for there will still however be coffee molecules and cream molecules combining. If we come back to human experience, when coach and coachee meet in a context, they will simultaneously experience the interplay and interaction of what is familiar to each of them and their sense of self to bring forth new experiences, perspectives and possibilities. We find the Gestalt idea of contact useful here as it allows individuals to pay attention to the degree to which they have fully become merged with context as in the case of confluence we described in Chapter 4, or are holding themselves and their individual sense of self separate from context. It opens up the possibility of examining the ways in which context is shaping individual experience and the extent to which this is chosen and optimal for the individual and the environment. Becoming conscious of these boundary dynamics is key to creating meaning and choice.

Figure 5.1 illustrates the overlapping boundaries in the coach-coachee-context situation. These boundaries, 1 (between coach and coachee), 2 (between coach and context) and 3 (between coachee and context), represent areas for individual and joint exploration in order to surface the particular nature and dynamics of each boundary, such as the degree of alignment or differentiation, and the assumptions that might be influencing relationship dynamics among the different parts. The central area where all boundaries overlap (4) represents the total situation that coach and coachee find themselves in. It is the area where the particular boundary dynamics of boundaries 1, 2 and 3 make themselves felt in the coaching relationship.

Multiple viewing angles

The following are a series of lenses or 'viewing angles' which illuminate only some of the many forces at work in shaping human experience, meaning making and patterns of behaviour. They are the different structures, socially constructed

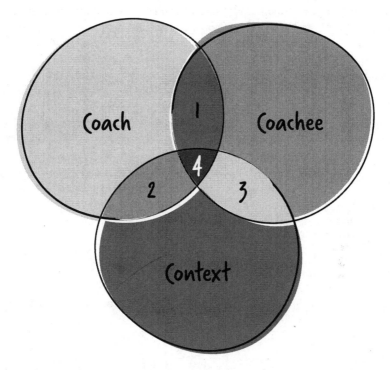

Figure 5.1 Overlapping boundaries in the coach-coachee-context constellation

forms, discourses and consensus realities held in individuals and social systems that influence and shape one another, determine individual experience, and which each of us has to navigate in the many different contexts in which we work and live. Each of these perspectives and the mental models they give rise to, will, to varying degrees, stand to influence feeling, thought and what happens in each unique coach-coachee-context constellation and the interventions coaches find themselves making or choosing to make. It is not possible to attend consciously to all these possible dimensions simultaneously, nor should we attempt to, for then we would have no inner space left to be in relationship with our clients, listen deeply and track the subtle processes and forces that arise in the uniqueness of each encounter. They are offered here to enable coaches to begin to open up to the multitude of forces potentially at work in all human contexts and whenever we come together to work with our clients. They represent an invitation to open up to the interconnectedness of multiple factors which combine in unique ways at any given moment, shaping perception, experience, meaning and action. From a Gestalt perspective this orientation to the wider field is fundamental to the process of collaborative inquiry at the heart of coaching and consulting (Francis, 2005; Parlett, 1997).

They can also be thought of as a series of lenses to support coaches to be alert and open to how a client might be constructing their particular reality, situation and place within it, as well as the dynamics of their relationship with the coach. They are simultaneously constructs which support meaning making, and enable questioning of whether a particular construction that might be revealing itself is in service of a client's well-being and success. They are not to be assumed to be truth, nor are they to be imposed on clients, but rather like maps, they provide a representation of the territory, while never being able to reflect the uniqueness, detail and changing contours of a particular landscape. Which of these (and other) forces might have bearing and relevance in any coach-coachee-context constellation can never be known in advance, but sensitive and effective coaches, through sensing and listening deeply to their clients and themselves, will be alert to how these fields of thinking might be informing a particular moment or situation and may bring them to awareness as a way of introducing catalytic diversity into the coaching conversation.

The following forces and systems of thought inevitably shape human interaction and meaning making, sometimes overtly, yet often they are subtle, and felt as an embodied sense of something. They are also inevitably implicated in the construction of coaching as a profession and each and every coaching conversation between coaches and their coachees.

Contract

The contract that is entered into between coach, coachee and context represen-tatives is a fundamental component influencing a specific coaching relationship and what can happen here in both overt and subtle ways. The contracting process itself, like the coaching process and possible outcomes, is shaped by a host of variables and can take many forms (see Chapter 10). The type of coaching, the mindsets of coaches and coachees, the context, public and private dynamics, all shape the forms that coaching might possibly take in a given situation at a given time. The art of coaching involves exploring the perspectives of those involved in the coaching engagement, introducing and negotiating differences and creating an appropriate frame for the work that can focus conversation. It also needs to hold the tension of coach, coachee and context requirements along with the spaciousness, reflexivity and flexibility to review the contract and re-contract on an ongoing basis, as more meaning is made by coach and coachee about the coachee's learning journey and the context she finds herself in.

Social, political, cultural

This is the territory of current socio-cultural trends, political and economic discourse in which coaching as a profession and individual coaching engagements are situated. The global financial crisis has in some quarters influenced not only the resources available for clients to make use of coaching, but coaching agendas are likely to be, among other things, informed by uncertainty and patterns of thinking and behaviour brought about by economic instability and the anxiety this gives rise to.

This is also the territory of ethnicity, gender discourse and power. Cultural trends in relation to the construction of ethnicity and difference, as well as gender, subtly find their ways into the coaching conversation. There is a wealth of evidence to show how ethnic and gender differences, along with power dynamics (Fletcher, 2001; King, 2012) shape the experience of clients and their organisations. Women clients of ours have often spoken of how behaviour they experience as aggressive in men in their organisations is construed as unprob-lematic and even desirable by the men, while they can be construed as aggressive and overly emotional by their male colleagues when they act in identical ways. Clients may well bring issues directly related to challenges of integration, inclusion and power into coaching. How different people, including coaches, construe their own sense of authority, agency and potency will also be informed by their experiences of gender and ethnicity and who is deemed to have power in the social and organisational systems they inhabit. Subtly and not so subtly these discourses, and the scripts they give rise to, infiltrate and shape individuals' experience, who they take themselves to be and what they have come to believe might be possible or equally be off limits for them.

How coaches and coachees think about agency and responsibility is also central to shaping the dynamics of the coaching relationship. From the individualistic perspective, agency tends to be assumed to reside in the individual who is seen to be the origin of action upon others or the environment. A more relational orientation sees agency (intentions, goals and actions) and impact to be a function of the interaction of individuals, their relationships and their contexts (McNamee and Gergen, 1999).

The family system constellations work of Bert Hellinger (Hellinger, 1998) focuses on surfacing the often invisible, yet palpable, forces at work in family systems, which give rise to individual feelings, behaviour and dis-ease. Hellinger's work has been taken up by organisation consultants and applied to examining organisation systems and the ways in which individual thought, experience and action are profoundly bound up with the system history and context in which people are living and working. A number of practitioners (Mackewn, 2014, 2015; Whittington, 2012) have taken the systemic constellations approach and applied it to coaching to enable coaches and coachees to surface and explore the multitude of forces shaping the action that coachees are able to take, and illuminating how, for individuals to expand in range for resolving complex organisational challenges, surfacing the wider forces at work and their impact in shaping individual experience is an essential dimension to changing individual behaviour.

Organisation context and dynamics

This is the territory of the particular organisation context in which coaching is taking place. The cultural patterns, thinking and behaviour that characterise the organisation will contribute to shaping the coach-coachee-context constellation. If the organisation is financially successful and buoyant the climate and pre-occupations of members are likely to be different than those of individuals whose organisations are failing or under imminent perceived 'threat' of hostile takeover.

The attitude to learning in an organisation is another important factor that can determine the uses coaches are put to, the purposes of the coaching engagement and what might be possible. In organisations that are characterised by extreme competitiveness, political jockeying and where deference to expertise abounds, coaching may be subtly and privately construed as remedial and a sign of weakness (in spite of public communication suggesting otherwise). In another organisation, coaching may be constructed as a privilege reserved only for high potential employees on leadership development programmes.

The ways in which coaches and coachees implicitly conceive of organisations is also significant here. In his seminal work, Morgan (1986, 1997) has set out a number of metaphors for organisations which capture many of the ways in which organisations have been and are conceived of still to this day. These include seeing the organisation as a machine, as nature, as a brain, as a psychic prison, and as a political system. In this book we have tended to concentrate on seeing organisations as social and complex fields of interaction. How we think of organisations and how we assume they operate, which is never likely to be a complete picture of how a particular organisation actually operates, will shape and determine how coachee and coach explore particular scenarios and think together about how to take action in the wider context.

Fisher, Rooke and Torbert (2003) point to how mental constructs and meaning making frameworks of organisation members govern the way organisations are conceived of and function. Drawing on the work of adult development researchers such as Cook-Greuter (2004), Kegan (1982) and Loevinger (1987) they conceive of a hierarchy of increasingly complex meaning making tendencies or 'action logics'. Less complex meaning making is often reliant on existing knowledge, processes and unquestioned assumptions, which then determine action. Increasingly complex meaning making is able to surface and question assumptions about theories in use, tolerate multiplicity of subjectivity and perspectives, evaluate existing strategies and experiment with the creation of new meaning and actions. The dominant action logic of an organisation and its members cannot but influence the way in which coaching is framed and what will be expected of it.

Life history, personhood of coach and coachee

The experience of early interactions, as we have seen, establishes deep and unique patterns of attachment, which in turn impact the capacity coach and coachee will have for relating, regulating anxiety, reflecting and making meaning. As subsequent life experiences are encountered, made sense of and mediated through the influence of early patterning, coach and coachee become the personalities they have become at the point at which they happen to meet. The personality styles of each, along with differences in action logics, life scripts, mental models, spiritual orientation, strengths and blind spots, all stand to inform the relationship, the negotiation of foci for the work, the way in which learning and development are facilitated and outcomes achieved. Coach training can develop the capacity in coaches for deep listening, bracketing of presuppositions, internal supervision and reflection in action and yet, at the same time, none of us can know what we do not know, or how we might subtly be impacted by coachees and their situations. We cannot predict the associations, feelings, thoughts, enactments and stuck moments that might arise and their potential relevance to the work. When this happens, it is important that coaches be able to reflect in the context of supervision on the subtle dance of co-emergence of experience as a result of two subjectivities in relationship. Furthermore, a relational orientation, which sees the dynamics of relating as central to how meaning is made, calls upon coaches to be willing to pay close attention to themselves and their experience moment by moment as well as that of their coachees. We shall explore these dynamics in more detail in the next two chapters.

Training frameworks, experience and organisational backgrounds of coach and coachee

The particular training and development histories of coaches and coachees represent another force which stands to shape interaction and the work that unfolds. Different professional paths, academic histories, teaching pedagogies and the philosophical assumptions embedded in them, all contribute to shaping the coach and coachee's orientation to knowledge and the facilitation of learning and change. Positivist scientific disciplines and research paradigms may orient coach and coachee towards logic and objectivity, whereas post-modern and relational ideas about the nature of reality, meaning and experience may orient coach and coachee more towards intersubjectivity and meaning as a negotiated and socially co-constructed phenomenon. It is inevitable that each orientation will inform how coach and coachee perceive, what stands out for them in their individual and co-constructed perceptual field, how each thinks and chooses to act. If viewed as a polarity, the assumptions embedded in positivism/modernism and those of post-modernism can both be seen to have different perspectives to offer. A positivist orientation might privilege identifying a clear and precise sense of direction and constructing a narrative about the path to achieving objectives and goals based on logic and existing principle. A post-modern orientation supports reflecting on the ways in which meaning is being made and allows for more of the subjective complexity of a given situation to be surfaced, thought about and adjusted to in order to work through or around obstacles.

Over adherence to either end of the continuum is also likely to limit perceptual possibilities and breadth of thinking and acting. Knowing which assumptions might be governing thinking and relating at any particular moment, and being able to shift viewing angles contributes to greater potential generativity. Different learning styles (Honey and Munford, 1992) and capacity for reflection (Mezirow, 1991) on the part of coach and coachee will also contribute to the meaning making processes that emerge in every coaching relationship. As coaches, the coaching profession, clients and their contexts evolve, we assume that coaches will need to draw on an increasing range of theoretical and practice orientations. From an integrative-relational perspective, the question becomes not so much simply 'what' does this particular coach have to offer, or 'how' does this particular coach work (as if this were fixed and identical with every client and context), but also how do we as coaches 'make use' of what we bring, in the uniquely different situations in which we work, in ways that clients might in turn be able to 'make use' of us to generate new insight and meaning appropriate to their needs and context requirements?

While coaches do need to have developed a robust theoretical model and related practice orientation, it can never be known in advance what will unfold between a coach and their coachee, what aspects of a coach's theoretical and practice orientation will emerge in use, how he might be challenged, stretched and confronted with the limitations of his current working model. For this reason coaches need also to cultivate the reflexivity, flexibility and openness to continuously evaluate their theory in use and expand it where necessary. Working models of the self, how change happens, the role and stance of the coach all stand to guide and inform thinking and action, and simultaneously need to be held lightly enough so that their usefulness in the uniqueness of each coach-coachee-context meeting can be monitored and evaluated. In this way coaches remain open to the mutually influencing relationship between theory and experience (theory shapes experience and vice versa) and the fact that they are not the same.

The experience of the present moment, reading and regulating exchanges

From a relational perspective, coach and coachee are seen to be involved in a relationship of reciprocal influence, communicating and making meaning in a process of informed gestures and responses. This calls for coaches to orient themselves to the present moment and pay attention to the quality of the relationship, connection, disconnection, the exchanges that take place and any particular patterns, stuckness or entanglements that might be occurring as coach and coachee interact. These patterns can be overt, but are often subtle and require skill and practice in order to be attuned to. From a relational perspective, these exchanges are seen as central to providing information about the work that is unfolding and are key to how meaning is made and change occurs in a one to one helping relationship. The degree to which coach and coachee can make overt use of these dynamics will contribute to shaping the form and direction coaching takes. We shall explore these 'micro' relational dynamics in more detail in the next two chapters.

Intervention

In the dance of reciprocal influence coaches will be making conscious and not so conscious choices about what to draw attention to, what questions to ask and how to respond to the coachee. Some coaches may be versed in particular theoretical frameworks for thinking about interventions such as Heron's Six Category Intervention Analysis (2001), which inclines practitioners to have clear intentions and strategies of execution. Others, such as those working with a Gestalt orientation, will be sensitised to finding and sharpening 'figures of interest' with the coachee, making use of their own experience and tracking closely which themes seem to have most energy associated with them for the coachee (Leary-Joyce, 2014). Some coaches may be more wedded to certain protocols and tools for intervening. All, however, will be being influenced in and out of conscious awareness by the multitude of forces at work in each coach-coachee-context constellation and the dance of reciprocal influence of the coaching relationship. Cavanagh (2006) sees client and coach as each being situated in their unique subjective system informed, among other things, by the different territories we have been discussing. In the complex adaptive conversation of the coaching relationship each gesture (verbal or otherwise) made by the coachee lands in the

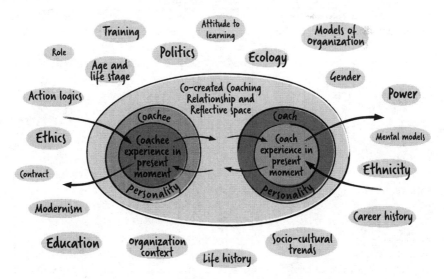

Figure 5.2 Multiple forces and factors influencing the gestures and responses of coach and coachee

field of the coach and her particular system of influences. On the basis of how the coach is impacted, she will make a response, which in turn lands in the field of the coachee and his system and generates another response and so on. Paying attention to the gestures and responses offers up much potential insight and information to be made use of in support of the coachee's learning and development.

Figure 5.2 shows how the individual experience of coach and coachee moment by moment is influenced by their individual gestures and responses, which in turn are mediated via their personalities and shaped as a result of the many forces in the wider context that each is situated in.

What we have attempted to show in this chapter are some of the different forces that contribute to shaping the coach-coachee-context situation, the coach-coachee relationship, the meaning that may arise in it and the gestures or interventions that a coach may make. The precise contours of each relationship and meaning can never be known in advance. As is the case with all maps, they are never the territory and so need to be held lightly and coupled with a phenomenological orientation to practice (See Chapter 8) in order that the uniqueness of every client's construction of meaning and experience can be discovered and attuned to. Having this in mind can go some way to supporting coaches to expand their range of meaning making frameworks and practice with different perceptual frames in service of helping clients to generate different and potentially more effective strategies in complex and challenging contexts.

The different forces we have set out will have a different pattern and organisation in both coach and coachee. What coachees say they want to achieve and how they think will be informed by the particular contours of their inner world and how it is shaped by the territories and discourses we have set out along with others. Similarly, how the coach views coaching, experiences the coachee and contributes to the coaching process will be shaped by her inner world and relationship to elements in the different force fields.

It is to this interaction and the relational interplay of the coaching relationship that we turn our attention in the next two chapters and how, in the reciprocally influencing gesture and response dynamics of the coaching conversation, the internal worlds and action orientations of both coach and coachee stand to be revealed and potentially changed.

Chapter 6

Intersubjectivity I

Understanding relationship dynamics from a developmental perspective

In this chapter we wish to explore in more depth the relational coaching process. We shall introduce a number of perspectives from developmental and neuro-biological research that are helpful for reflecting on the micro dynamics and interactions of the coaching relationship and for considering their potential role in fostering collaboration and facilitating change.

The implicit and explicit dimensions of relationship and interaction

Current developmental and neurobiological research points to the crucial importance for change practitioners to understand the interface between what is termed the explicit verbal level of relating, the domain of the 'narrative', and the implicit, non-verbal, somatic embodied level of relating – how it feels to be with an other person moment by moment. This research demonstrates that implicit relational knowing underscores all relational interactions as a constantly present factor between coach and coachee, informing our experience and construction of whatever overt narrative we are engaged in.

The Boston Change Process Study Group (2010) describe 'forms of relational meaning' which involve the interface between 'implicit relational knowing' and the 'reflective verbal domain'. Implicit relational knowing, the embodied knowl-edge each of us has developed of 'how to be with others', influences our intimate reactions that are not routinely translated into language, because we simply experience these responses as part of what we 'know' and experience inside ourselves about how to react. It is this which gives a felt sense of getting on with an other, or conversely, feeling as if something is not quite right in a particular relationship.

This process is not experienced in conscious awareness, as these responses are not translated into language or other symbolic forms. The reflective verbal domain of experience, however, involves the creation of the narratives that give meaning to our direct lived experience, the labels we attach to felt experiences. These two domains develop, co-exist and interact with one another throughout our lives. Neuroscience research (Cozolino 2006; 2013) has amply demonstrated that our brain is not a static organ, it continually changes in response to environmental stimuli and different challenges, and as coaches we can support coachees to address such challenges in the context of an empathic, collaborative and accepting relationship that pays attention to the crucial interface between the implicit and the explicit.

A coachee who is anxious in the face of a significant challenge, and whose anxiety is in part created by the ways in which he is making meaning about his situation and his role in it, will stand to be influenced not just by the coach's support in reframing the client's narrative at the cognitive level, but in large part by the coach's welcoming, calm, attuned, responsive and reflective manner. Should the coach also be prone to anxiety and move quickly to finding solutions, working hard to drive a change of belief in the coachee, the coachee may well pick this up *implicitly* as a sign of danger, hinting that the situation really is as awful as the coachee believes it to be. He may get the impression that anxiety cannot be tolerated, contained and thought about, but has to be expelled into activity and finding a quick fix. A coachee may also conclude at the level of cognition that there is something not OK about him on the basis of the coach's reactivity to the situation and urgency in trying to change it. Consulting practices, which intentionally portray organisation challenges as worse or more dangerous than they actually might be exploit this dynamic to increase client anxiety and foster greater dependency on the consultants who can then be cast in the role of expert-saviours. Coachees can, however, learn to slow down and reflect by being in the presence of a different quality of energy, psychological spaciousness and calm reflexivity as embodied by their coach, which in turn can support more ownership of responsibility, informed and improved decision-making and action.

The boundaries between the two domains of the implicit and the explicit are permeable and both lead to an embodied sense of our experience of others. We can 'learn' new behaviour consciously through reflecting on our familiar patterns of acting in the world and taking the initiative to change these, a significant domain of much coaching theory to date. We can also 'learn' at the implicit level through our relationship with others, which comes more into focus in a relational orientation to coaching and includes the quality of the coach's presence, tone of voice and attunement to the client's inner experience. At the explicit verbal level coaches can provide an environment where support is balanced with challenge, so enabling the coachee to challenge their own assumptions and existing narratives about their capabilities, work contexts and relationships with colleagues. These can then be reconstructed in the light of new perspectives emerging with the coach through the interaction of felt experience and the ability to think about it.

As the implicit level of learning happens below the level of conscious awareness, we absorb this 'learning' as we interact with people. Through experiencing the acceptance, understanding, empowerment and collaboration conveyed in a coaching relationship, a coachee will be gaining a new experience of relating at both these interacting levels of experience. If the coach-coachee relationship conveys new implicit ways of regulating anxiety, provides attention to what is arising in here-and-now experience, and sensitivity to feelings, then a coachee will be impacted and changed by these processes without necessarily consciously reflecting on this learning (see the example in Chapter 3). If he is encouraged to reflect on his emotional embodied process, how he is feeling, and put words to this experience, he will integrate his learning at both explicit and implicit levels.

This means that for the coach it is vital to realise that it is not only the words we say but how we say these words that conveys our relational energy. The tone of our voice, the rhythm and textures of our language, how we sit and move in the process of communicating, the melody of our voice (prosody) which Stern (1998) has referred to as 'vitality affects' (p. 53). We respond to these processes below the level of conscious awareness, so a focus on bodily responses and somatic awareness can bring us in touch with more of our own feelings, embodied experience and profound human need to be truly understood by an 'other'.

As meaning emerges from the interaction of these two levels of communication, if there is a dysjunction between them, those participating in the relationship will 'sense' this incongruence without necessarily being able to articulate the 'reasons' for their discomfort. When coaching, we may for example experience our coachee talking in an animated and vivacious manner about how all is going very well, whereas at the same time we are aware of a slight hesitation and tentativeness about the eyes of the person, a sagging of the shoulders. Sensitively drawing attention to this bodily process where possible can gradually enable the person to recognise aspects of his experience he may be denying for the sake of 'putting on a brave face' as he tries to align with what he imagines might be expected in his organisation. Surfacing this particular construction is a vital step in coachees being able to begin to accurately assess their personal and professional challenges as they experience them, and find the specific support they may actually need to face them squarely and creatively.

Effective and generative dialogue between coach and coachee is also co-created at both levels of experience. We grasp the intention of the communication intuitively and experience this in a felt embodied manner without easily being able to put this into words. So a coachee may say 'I felt my first coach didn't "get me", but the second one just understood immediately what I needed'. In this second example there is likely to have been more congruence between the implicit and explicit levels of communication, whereas the first coach may have said the 'right' things but did not 'inhabit' his own expression. This could be as a result of the coach wanting to communicate or sell an approach or strategy at a conceptual level, perhaps with a slight evangelical enthusiasm, and without taking the time to attune to the coachee and his experience. This is also a familiar risk for coaches if we become overly and prematurely fixated on outcomes. We might hold a tight task focus, deploying a series of techniques, while losing touch with the felt sense of being with the coachee and how we are responding to him or her moment by moment. Over the years a number of our clients have commented on what seems paradoxical to them (but makes sense in the context of working with attention to implicit and explicit domains of experience), that they do not feel as 'pushed' as they have felt with other coaches, but that they nonetheless experience that they are learning much about themselves, developing greater reflection and meaning making capacity about the challenging situations they find themselves in, developing more refined skills and expanding their repertoires for acting differently.

This embodied experience of relationship is also supported by the neuro-biological research on how 'mirror neurons' (which we referred to in the previous chapter) are linked to our process of social identification. By a non-verbal, embodied process of communication referred to as 'embodied simulation' (Ammaniti and Gallese, 2014, p. 15) people 'learn' how to be with others through 'mutual resonance'.

When we are in the presence of an other, we are able, through the firing of our mirror neurons to experience something of what the other person is experiencing, even if we do not actively engage in the same behaviours. Embodied simulation mediates and is key to our capacity to share the meaning of actions, intentions, feelings and emotions with others, thus grounding our identification with, and connectedness to, others. In this respect it is central to the experience of empathy and attuning to one another's experience (Gallese, 2001, 2003a, 2003b). This is a 'prerational' space in which we do not reflect but simply are impacted by and absorb experience. In this way, as children, we learn how to be with others and to 'read' their intentions. This is a non-conscious process in which we share implicitly what it is to be human. This process continues to be part of our experience in adult life. In this way we develop a world of shared meaning. It is this principle that supports the need for coaches to be more sensitive and attuned to the felt sense of a coachee's experience in their context, broadening their orientation and practice beyond the cognitive domain of individual beliefs and assumptions to include more of the coachee's emotional and felt experience.

This can be challenging given the dominance of cognition in organisational life, and we are not advocating that coaches should go hunting for emotion and felt experience. Yet it is becoming increasingly necessary to pay attention to a fuller human experience in the face of complex situations and challenges that cannot simply be thought through and controlled through the application of familiar mechanisms, existing strategies, logic and reason (Watkins, 2014). Rather they need to be thought *and* 'felt' through, and the relationship between feeling and thinking made more explicit. In this way cognition and the feeling of things can be brought into dialogue and enrich the sources of information available to a coachee about her own experience, the context she is working in, how she is being impacted and how she might experiment with new and creative responses where these are called for.

This means that for coaches, the sense of our presence and our way of being with the coachee will be as important as the words we speak. The coachee will have an intuitive, embodied sense of the congruence between these two levels of their experience of the coaching. The coachee may express this in words like 'I felt immediately at ease with you', 'I sense that you have my interest at heart even when you challenge me' and 'It was as though you understood what I was experiencing even though I was struggling to put this into words – I now have a much better sense of how this is affecting me and what I need to be doing differently'.

The challenge for coaches, given the dominance of cognitive, explicit and individualistic assumptions underpinning much coaching theory and practice to date, is to accept that this level of communication is always at work in our coaching relationships. Engaging in personal reflection, supervision and mindfulness or meditative practice will support us to reflect and maintain our own authenticity in life and in our coaching practice. It is not only what I do or say, but how I embody what I say, that will resonate with the coachee and stand to facilitate learning and change at many levels.

Affect regulation

'Affect regulation' has been the subject of much neurobiological research of the last decade (Schore and Schore, 2008; Schore, 2009) and refers to the capacity to be aware of, reflect on and make mature choices about expressing our emotions appropriately in the present with due regard to the impact this may have on others. In the process of growing up, we may have learnt to repress certain basic emotions and states (like anger, sadness or vulnerability) in order to avoid rejection, which means we do not learn to experience, make use of and express such emotions in a mature adult way. Subsequently these emotions may 'burst out' in an unregulated manner which jeopardises our relationships and our capacity to engage in generative and collaborative conversations at work.

Emotions are a vital source of information about how we are making sense of and responding to a particular situation and, at the same time, we need to guard against being overwhelmed by them so that they become a source of non-reflective emotionality and behaviour that is impulsively acted out rather than consciously chosen.

In the current neurobiological and child development literature the terms 'affect regulation' and 'affect dysregulation' (Schore, 2003) refer to a person's development of this capacity to regulate their own emotions both internally through awareness and reflection, and in expressing emotions effectively in interaction with others. As we set out earlier, this capacity for appropriate self and interactive regulation (Beebe and Lachmann, 2002) in establishing and maintaining relationships is developed through interaction with a self-regulating other, including parents and significant caregivers, who can manage their own arousal and respond appropriately, in the course of healthy development.

However, given the reality of human beings, even if we grew up in 'an average expectable environment' (Winnicott, 1965) with ordinary 'good-enough' parenting, we may still have developed certain patterns of regulation that do not always serve us well.

Beebe and Lachmann (1998) point out that some people tend to under-regulate their emotions while others tend to over-regulate, and sometimes people shift from one to another under pressure. People who under-regulate tend to let their emotions 'overflow' by, for example, having outbursts of rage or anxiety, while people who over-regulate often show no expression of emotion at all in situations where others feel moved. They point out that the middle of the range has been shown to predict 'secure attachment' (Bowlby, 1969; 1973) where the person can freely choose their own level of energy in an encounter, and move along the range as suits the particular situation, whereas being 'stuck' at either extreme can be problematic. As a coach it is important to take into account the coachee's style of regulation at the particular point of a meeting and attune accordingly if we wish to establish a connection supportive of effective work. Furthermore, these perspectives on attachment and affect regulation can be useful in understanding the relational patterns coachees may display with the coach and those they describe with peers, superiors and subordinates. This offers ways of improving regulation and range of response where necessary.

For working with clients, Beebe and Lachmann (2002) suggest a number of strategies, although these are tentative suggestions and by no means exhaustive: matching or tracking the coachee to convey empathy and understanding, referred to as 'joining'; either raising the energy if the coachee is very dampened down, or soothing if the person is overcome with emotion, referred to as 'altering'; or maintaining an unvarying level of energy if the person seems very cautious of connection, referred to as 'neutrality'. These are important strategies to consider in terms of attuning to coachees in order to 'reach' the person on an implicit relational level as we move on with the explicit coaching contract.

Widening the 'window of tolerance'

Personal and professional change in the complex, unpredictable and intersubjective environments many clients work in depends on being able to widen the 'window of tolerance' (Siegel, 1999). In the face of the challenges of the VUCA world, coachees often need to manage their feelings of anxiety and uncertainty, be willing to take calculated risks and experiment with new behaviours and conversations. Data are often partial and coachees will not be able to predict the outcomes of their actions. Siegel (1999) describes the window of tolerance as the window each of us has within which various intensities of emotional arousal can be processed without disrupting the functioning of the person. It can be narrow or wide, and each of us will differ in relation to what emotions or stressors we can tolerate and those which take us out of the window. One coachee may be able to tolerate a great amount of ambiguity and go on thinking and choosing how to respond. For another, even a little uncertainty might be experienced as overwhelming and intolerable, leading to rigidity of thinking, a narrow range of action or automatic responses that are not thought through. Another coachee may be able to easily and comfortably tolerate angry and aggressive behaviour in her boss, whereas for another, a simple confused frown on his manager's face might be enough to fill him with anxiety and concern about reputation and future career prospects.

If an experience pushes us outside our window of tolerance we may fall into chaos on the one hand termed 'hyperarousal', or rigidity and depression on the other referred to as 'hypoarousal'. Hyperarousal results from the sympathetic nervous system's response to stress by increasing energy consuming processes like increased heart rate and respiration, as might be required in a fight or flight response to danger. Hypoarousal is as a result of the action of the parasympathetic nervous system increasing energy conserving processes such as decreased heart rate, respiration, numbness and shutting down the mind, as might be required for freeze, submit and feigned death (as seen in the animal kingdom) responses to threat. Although we are unlikely to be dealing with threats to actual survival with our coachees, research into trauma (Levine, 2010; Ogden *et al.*, 2006) has shown that the brain is not always able to differentiate between degrees of risk, particularly when an individual is out of their window of tolerance. Many of the more stressful challenges and responsibilities coachees face can trigger these responses to varying degrees which can have a direct bearing on a coachee's ability to realistically assess a situation they are in and make use of the coaching conversation to reflect and generate effective options for action.

Stress, anxiety, emotions and cognitions all mutually influence one another (Ogden *et al.*, 2006). Negative thoughts can give rise to anxiety and vice versa. When leaning towards hyperarousal, coachees may be inclined to think in rigid and absolute ways, they may be prone to catastrophic thinking, magnifying and escalating the negative implications of possible scenarios and options. They may want to rush into action and will not be able to slow down to reflect and make more informed meaning about their situation (as often happens with quick, reactive, and often later regretted, responses to challenging emails!). They may feel overly responsible, while also doubting their ability. Similarly, clients who may be more hypoaroused will seem very flat in energy. They may appear overwhelmed and helpless, unable to engage with their coach and the coaching conversation.

From a relational perspective, being able to monitor moment by moment the extent to which a coachee is in their window of tolerance or not is a rich source of information about his capacity to reflect, be flexible, curious and open to experimentation both in relation to the coaching conversation and whatever challenges he might be facing in the wider organisation. A narrow window of tolerance constricts our capacity to process information, remain receptive, reflective, creative, aware and consciously choose our responses.

Affect regulation and meaning making

The Boston Change Process Study Group (2010) have identified the co-regulation of affect and the co-creation of meaning as two key types of learning that develop throughout the lifespan and are central in supporting the capacity to respond to increasing ambiguity and complexity. Coaches can enable coachees to widen their window of tolerance by helping them directly to manage their levels of stress and arousal through, if skilled in this area, teaching tools and techniques such as mindfulness practices. In addition to this, in the coaching conversation, coaches can enable coachees to remain in their window of tolerance through the quality of the coach's own energy, presence and responses. In this respect, coaches can offer a form of interactive regulation in the same way that original caregivers can enable young children to feel soothed and calmed which is critical to developing the capacity for regulating emotions in adulthood. Key to this process is the coach's capacity to manage his own state and widen his own window of tolerance in order to remain present, receptive and responsive in the face of a client who might be anxious, demanding and rigid in their thinking and action. The more a coachee is supported through interactions with the coach to manage arousal and remain reflective, the more he will widen the window of tolerance and so be able to increase tolerance of stress without sacrificing his capacity to reflect, make meaning and respond flexibly. This learning then becomes available to the coachee outside of the coaching room whenever he finds himself in challenging and uncertain situations.

Free flowing conversation

A central question from a relational perspective is whether coach and coachee are able to conduct a free-flowing conversational exchange? This may seem a very obvious question, yet we will have experienced many people who talk and talk without giving the other person any space to respond so that as the listener you begin to feel redundant. If a client behaves like this in the wider organisational context, they are likely to experience and contribute to communication challenges that impede effective functioning. Lee and Martin (1991) make a number of observations about conversational rhythms that have come out of developmental research, namely 'alternating and coactive speech patterns', (p. 301). 'Alternating rhythms' are characteristic of a conversation in which people take turns to speak, each giving the other the opportunity to respond before continuing. With this pattern the turn of the other is respected and granted space. This pattern is much more conducive to generating understanding, exploring different perspectives and collaborating to make meaning in relationship with others so necessary in complex organisational contexts. This process is originally learnt by the child in interaction with a caring and responsive other so that the adult is easily able to engage in mutual conversational exchange. However, the child may have been 'talked at' without being given much opportunity for a response; a situation, alas, that is often repeated in organisational contexts where the person in power may leave little space for dialogue, or where leadership team members jockey to assert their individual perspectives with no interest in the perspectives of others.

'Coactive rhythms' refer to moments of heightened connection when both parties may speak or react at the same time, or laugh, or be moved to tears, or be angry, or remain deeply and respectfully silent. It is a point at which both parties 'join' in a special exchange and there is a deep sense of meeting. These experiences can have an almost magical quality of sharing, a moment of meeting as two equal human beings.

A coachee once reported how she felt as if her manager was distant and seemingly uninterested in her and her work. She confronted him, and, in a rather unconsidered and animated way, told him how angry she was and how she thought he had simply not considered her in making a particular decision that was going to have a significant and challenging impact in her department. His unexpected, undefended and genuine reply, 'Oh, I'm really sorry, I completely underestimated how important my decision and our relationship is to you' took her by surprise, and she saw him in a new way as a person of sensitivity. She also learnt from this exchange the importance of being able to stay reflective and choose a more respectful response as was demonstrated by her manager's response to her angry outburst. They subsequently developed a healthy and productive collaborative working relationship. This was an example of a coactive moment that enriched the relationship.

Mentalisation and the development of the reflective function

In current infant development literature there is a central focus on the concept of mentalisation, which describes an individual's capacity to be aware of the feelings, reactions and ways of experiencing the world of other people, as being different from his or her own. This is seen as a developmental milestone when the child is able to 'read' and interpret the minds of others and appreciate the different beliefs, feelings, attitudes, desires, hopes, knowledge, imagination, along with the intentions, plans, insincerity, deceit and pretence of others with whom they are in a relationship (Fonagy *et al.*, 2002). This is also referred to as the 'reflective function' or the development of a 'theory of mind' (Fonagy, 1997). What is of interest to us as coaches is that for some adults this may not be as well developed as for others. There are certainly people who generally can really struggle to see the perspectives of others. Assisting coachees to develop and/or strengthen their reflective function we see as one of the most important tasks of the coach, particularly in the context of the VUCA world. It is key to supporting 'vertical' development, expanding leaders' mental constructs and action logics (Fisher, Torbert and Rooke, 2003; Laloux, 2014) in order for them to manage greater complexity and paradox in their contexts. This capacity to take a meta-perspective on a situation and appreciate the self in relation to others forms the basis of effective leadership in complex contexts. It underlies the capacity to appreciate the impact that we have on others given our styles of relating, and involves being able to tolerate and think about the multiple subjectivities of those with whom we interact, seek to engage and lead.

It is also a feature of most of our lives that, at times of stress when we are pushed to the edges of our 'window of tolerance' by the unexpected, or events we experience as overwhelming, we may lose our capacity to reflect and to appreciate the complexities of a situation. Earlier we described how our thinking and behaviour can be affected if anxiety takes us out of our unique individual window of tolerance. At that point we lose our perspective on the event/interaction and may feel 'persecuted' by others or move into 'persecuting' them, with no capacity at that moment to appreciate the perspective of the other. Michael Carroll (Carroll and Gilbert, 2011) refers to this as 'zero reflection'.

Whenever we are working with a coachee who is at the edge of her window of tolerance, and has temporarily lost the capacity for mentalisation, it is important to stay with the here-and-now dynamic of the relationship and attune to the person's state in order to to facilitate a return to conditions supportive of the learning process. This may include naming the fact that the coach has noticed the coachee moving into a more anxiety-based pattern of feeling, thinking and acting. However, it can also happen on occasions that we as coaches revert to 'zero reflection' under challenge or stress. Then, as soon as we become aware that this has happened, it is necessary for us to re-invoke our reflective capacity. For example, we may find ourselves in a situation where we feel irritated because 'this coachee is resistant to learning, and is so obstinate about his own point of view that he will not use my skill as a coach!' At which point we are actually replicating what we are 'seeing' in the coachee!

As we practice and develop our own reflective skills we may gradually learn to catch ourselves moving into this non-reflective stance at times of stress and, through internal supervision and 'reflection-in-action' (Carrol and Shaw, 2013; Hawkins and Shohet, 2012; Schon, 1983), be able once more to exercise our choice and responsibility in the situation. We can also support ourselves and our clients through mindfulness practices designed to support a slowing down of non-reflective reactivity, putting a pause between stimulus and response. Our early developmental processes often set the scene for the coach's and coachee's present moment adult capacity to be in relationship, interact fruitfully with others, process thoughts, adjust to the requirements of the environment, in order to engage in productive ongoing learning. It is for this reason that a relational orientation to coaching involves coaches paying close attention to their experience of being in relationship with their coachees and learning about their own familiar patterns, as well as changing them as part of the process of being with an other. This is one of the most challenging as well as deeply satisfying aspects of this orientation.

The influence of each individual's organising principles on the coaching relationship

Patterns of relating that people have developed over time will be evident in their interactions with others in the present including with colleagues and the coach.

These patterns of interaction will be characteristic of the person's way of approaching relationships. Although such repetitive patterns have been labeled in different ways in the psychoanalytic literature such as 'transference' and 'counter-transference', we prefer the term 'organising principles' used in intersubjectivity theory to describe these 'maps' of the world, based on prior experience, that shape a person's perception of events in the present (Stolorow and Atwood, 1992). Our organising principles have often been powerfully influenced by our early experiences in our family, at school, in our culture of origin, but later influences may be equally powerful. They are ways of dealing with the world and, if laid down under stressful or traumatic circumstances, may lead to defensive ways of being in adulthood that interfere with effective communication with people around us. Because our organising principles are so much part of our experience, and operate largely below the level of conscious awareness, we may not stop to question the implicit assumptions that may inform these and 'believe' our view of 'reality' to be the only one!

We may have had rewarding, or disturbing experiences that powerfully impacted on our ways of relating to others and shape our subsequent interactions. While we all have these characteristic ways of approaching others, these patterns are also being constantly changed and updated as we meet new situations and people, provided that we are open to this moment-by-moment learning process. So, although our organising principles may be firmly set in our experience and reinforced by subsequent events, the challenge for the coach is to facilitate the coachee to become aware of what reactions may be unhelpful in the present and choose different options to achieve a desired outcome. This will involve, at its best, an updating of organising principles that widens the person's repertoire and creates greater flexibility, opening up new possibilities.

For the coach it is important to be asking 'How does the coachee organise the relationship with me?' and 'How do my organising principles configure my perception of this coachee?' In the coaching relationship we are in an inter-subjective matrix in which we are co-constructing a relationship to which both parties contribute moment-by-moment and over time as we develop a working alliance with each coachee. The organising principles of both in this collaborative relationship will shape the nature of the interaction. These processes operate largely out of conscious awareness for us so that we are often inclined to assume that our experience matches that of others around us. How often do we hear: 'I thought that as a team we all agreed that . . .' or 'It is obvious to everyone in the department that . . .?'

There will also be certain cultural norms embedded in our accepted view of behaviour (see the previous chapter), which may only come to light when we meet a 'contradiction'. People who have moved from one culture to another, or who work across cultures in global organisations, will need to develop a sensitivity to these cultural nuances. A response that from one perspective may be viewed as understated and lacking in passion, may from someone else's cultural perspective be viewed as a composed and well modulated response! Similarly an interaction that from one perspective is viewed as 'brash and tactless' may be viewed from another as 'forthright and honest, calling a spade a spade!' So as coaches we need to sensitise ourselves and our coachees to these different styles of expression and help them explore and question their underlying assumptions as to their universal validity.

Underlying scripts or schemas that influence perception of events and others

Researchers have also drawn attention to how certain principles may coalesce into a particular way of constellating all our relational experience. The term 'core interpersonal schema' (Beitman and Saveanu, 2005) has been used to describe a pattern of assumptions that informs our perception and assessment of events in relation to others. This schema is based on our early experiences of carers and then modified by subsequent experience. Our schemas (which contribute to making up the personality as set out in Chapter 2) influence our perception of others and how we interpret their 'motives' at an implicit level. Transactional Analysis refers to these schemas as our 'script', our personal 'story' about the world created out of our early experiences, responses and meaning made from them, which may colour much of our subsequent expectations and responses (Berne, 1972). Because we are largely unaware of such scripts or schemas, since they operate below the level of conscious awareness, we may assume 'that this is the way the world is' and that there is no possibility for different perspectives, possibilities and choices.

We ourselves do not take a deterministic view of these processes, since we believe that such 'maps' can be changed and updated throughout life in response to new experiences. However, this constitutes a challenge because as humans we may wish to stick with what is familiar, has worked in the past and feels central to our identity, even where this might limit our ability to function effectively. The challenge is to accept the concept of 'lifelong learning' linked to an active ongoing engagement in the change process.

This stance is very much supported by neuroscience that has demonstrated that new synaptic connections can be formed throughout life, that we are 'never too old to learn' if we are open to the challenge (Schwartz and Begley, 2002). However, it requires the development of our reflective function for us to become aware of ourselves and become aware of choices and responsibility. This is the challenge and vital function of the coach – to facilitate this process of developing awareness and learning. We see that the increased emphasis in coaching on processes like 'mindfulness' practice, developing self-reflexivity, increasing 'emotional intelligence', regulating arousal and transformational learning are aimed at raising our awareness of our scripts and schemas and making more creative choices that we may not previously have considered.

Krantz (1993) has examined in detail ways in which early relational templates associated with parent figures can find their ways into interactions between superiors and subordinates in organisational hierarchies. They can colour relationship dynamics and conversations inhibiting or facilitating understanding and effective communication. Given that from a relational and complexity perspective interactions and patterns of communication are key to how individuals function and organise in their particular enterprise, surfacing, understanding and re-working these schemas is key to individual and organisational change.

The evolving self – The development of the 'self-in-relationship' with relevance to coaching

Coaching at its best offers a safe, trusting, sufficiently novel and appropriately unsettling relationship in which the coachee can begin to address the challenges that he brings to coaching in a non-judgemental context. Following Buber (1965b) and the core tenets of Gestalt (Hycner and Jacobs, 1995) we believe in the importance of genuine dialogue, where coach and coachee engage in an experience of meeting as two subjectivities in a particular context and time, and where there is a commitment to welcoming and allowing the uniqueness and fullness of each to be present and available for the encounter.

It is important for the coach to balance support and confrontation in a manner and at a level that the coachee can accept at both a cognitive and emotional level and use to build his reflective capacities. Coaching offers a unique opportunity for such growth and extension of awareness because we are generally working with successful adults who come to us to promote their professional development and skills in the workplace. At the heart of this process of growth is creating a learning environment and supporting coachees to reflect in-depth on their interactions with self and others in order to achieve their goals.

We are born into relationship and develop our sense of self worth in relation to others as we develop and grow. Coaching potentially offers an enriched environment, an open, honest and trusting space in which the coachee can reflect on his outdated patterns of relating and make the changes that will enrich his interactions with self and others.

The development of self-in-relationship will occur at both implicit, non-verbal levels of communication between two people, and at the verbal level of interaction where the issues brought to coaching will be overtly addressed. At its best it enables the coachee to strengthen her sense of self, look again at the narrative of her experience and develop new perspectives that enhance her options in the workplace and in the world. Cozolino (2013) reinforces that the quality of the emotional connection and the emotional resonance between practitioner and client, coach and coachee is central to this process of change and growth.

It is to this relational process that we turn our attention in the following chapter.

Chapter 7

Intersubjectivity 2

The co-creation of the coaching relationship, meaning and change

In this chapter we move from a developmental perspective and how this might inform the coaching relationship to considering the dynamics of the relationship as they unfold between coach and coachee from an intersubjective perspective.

The dynamics of the co-created coaching relationship – An intersubjective perspective

As we described earlier, we see the coaching relationship as a two-person endeavour to which both participants contribute and to which both bring their own 'organising principles' based on their past experience of relationships. When two people come together, they bring to the encounter their own inner experience as this is embedded in their history, contexts and the meanings they have constructed from these. This experience comes to be expressed in the present context in a continual flow of reciprocal mutual influence (Stolorow and Atwood, 1992) and each is shaped by the other in this interaction. Through being open to considering these dynamics, coach and coachee stand, therefore, potentially to learn much about the influence of past experiences, meaning and context on their 'here and now' patterns of interaction and surface the assumptions and meanings that underpin them. Learning about how each is and acts in the world reveals itself in the relationship and offers information about each, their relationship and the impacts of social and contextual forces on their meaning making.

Authentic meeting

The primary aim of the collaboration between coach and coachee is to engage in a creative, spontaneous dialogue that allows for new experiences and meaning to emerge, which in turn shape future action. The quality of the relational climate and interactions between coach and coachee are key to creating conditions in which learning and change can occur. Moments of meeting in an authentic encounter between two human beings are central to effective coaching as these 'I-Thou' moments (Buber, 1958) can facilitate contact and change (Hycner, 1993; Hycner and Jacobs, 1995). This is further supported by the research of

Beebe and Lachmann (2002) who developed the concept of 'heightened affective moments' as being important in the change process.

Moments of emotional meeting may involve a humorous exchange, the sharing of a deeply felt disappointment, sadness or loss, moments of intense joy and moments of anxiety, stress and tension. Moments of meeting that involve anger or distress may upset the free-flow of the conversation. What is important here is that these moments often mark stages in the change process, and if reflected upon, can lead to new learning at a cognitive, emotional and somatic level. Berne (1966) observed that when confrontation occurs the person may respond with a 'thoughtful silence or an insightful laugh' (p. 235). The thoughtful silence may lead to change or the person may simply revert to their previous position; however, the insightful laugh usually signals 'a decisive cathectic shift' (p. 235), meaning that the psychic energy previously bound up in maintaining the inconsistency that the confrontation challenges is released. It usually, therefore, marks a shift for the client that is often enduring. This premise seems also to be relevant in our coaching practice. An ill-timed confrontation with little relational connection between coach and coachee can lead to reinforcing a fixed position; whereas the timely use of humour 'laughing with rather than laughing at' can lead to an awareness of a fixed, repetitive process that opens up new possibilities.

A coachee had worked for some time with her coach on her believing and feeling that she lacked in capability and authority in the face of a new challenging role. The client had come to see how her tendency towards self-doubt undermined her and she had come a long way in developing a more realistic assessment of her capacity. She had discovered that she found it helpful to draw on the support of her coach and a couple of trusted colleagues to restore her sense of efficacy when anxiety and doubt crept in. This was a significant development, as in the past she had tended to retreat from contact with others when doubting herself thereby reinforcing a sense of limitation and failure. At one session the coach arrived to find her in the grip of doubt and harsh self-criticism. As the coach listened to her litany of imagined failings and what had been happening in the time since their last meeting, the client began to settle and calm through being in the presence of the non-judgemental, spacious and responsive attitude of her coach who was genuinely curious to know how this increase in doubt had come about. It soon became apparent that, in the face of a very demanding workload, the client had isolated herself from her sources of support and reality testing, in spite of knowing the value she derived from these relationships. Given the quality of the relationship the coach felt he had with the client, and knowing she was a fan of Tolkien's Lord of the Rings and had just been to see the film with her son, he said 'what strikes me is that left to your own devices you can still take yourself off to the land of Mordor!' (– a barren land inhabited by demons!). The client laughed out loud in recognition, and coach and coachee were able to share in the lightness and truth for the client of the statement. This marked a shift for the coachee who, thereafter, was more aware of her need to reach out for support, particularly at times of increased pressure at work.

Co-responsibility

In a relational orientation to coaching, a fundamental working assumption is that each member of the dyad is seen as needing to take responsibility for his or her own part in the coaching process, adopting an orientation of co-responsibility. The role of coach may bring with it certain professional and ethical responsibilities, and the coachee (provided no pressure has been exerted by the coach) is the only one who can be responsible for how he chooses to make use of the coaching in his context. In the present moment dance of the coaching relationship, however, each is ultimately responsible for how each interacts, gestures and responds. Each is responsible for what comes to mind, what emotions, meanings and possibilities occur to each and how these are spoken out (or not) and responded to. The relationship is located in an intersubjective context in which two 'subjects' are in communication to create an effective learning environment. Each has responsibility for the sense that is being made, how it is being made, what each is feeling and how each is participating in the exchange. This is particularly relevant at times of challenge, stuckness or heightened emotions, where it is important that coach and coachee are able to find ways to name what is occurring between them and examine this for what it might have to say about the relationship, the perspectives and actions of each and the ways the work is unfolding.

Co-emergence

From a relational perspective, we are always located in the wider context of the organisation, and indeed the world around us. Our ever-developing sense of self will be influenced by all the factors in the field, of which the coaching relationship forms an important component (see Chapter 5). As we discussed in earlier chapters, our sense of self and our various self-states are constantly in an emergent state, being organised, constructed, deconstructed and reconstituted in our interactions with others in context (Cavicchia, 2009; Philippson, 2001). In this way coaching can provide a person with a space to explore how they are constructing themselves, acknowledge and examine ways in which context might be supporting or inhibiting them, access hidden parts of themselves that may be discounted or denied, integrate these into their self-concept in a manner that can achieve greater self-coherence, extend their range and repertoire of responses and, thereby, enhance their performance.

As we set out in the previous chapter, the process of change occurs at both the implicit embodied, non-verbal level of experience, and at the reflective-verbal level of interaction (Boston Change Process Study Group, 2010). At best these two domains of experience are congruent with one another so that we experience the other as genuine, sincere and open in interactions. This 'implicit relational knowing' (Boston Change Process Study Group, 2008) is at its best conveyed to a client by a coach who is able to be congruent. In the coach-coachee dialogue we pay attention to the total communication and its intention 'in one intuitive grasp', we sense into both the verbal and felt sense of interactions between coach and coachee, and it 'is this gestalt that gives out the multiple meanings that can shift and change over ongoing and repeated contemplation' (p. 145). As coaches we notice what we observe, how we are impacted, and any inconsistencies between what we hear, see and feel. Inevitably, since we are human and cannot fully know what may be out of conscious awareness but which still makes itself felt, there will be disjunctions between the implicit and the verbal levels of interaction. If there is a disjunction between what is felt and what is said, then the listener (whether coach or coachee) will sense this at some, often embodied, level of experience, and realise that he is dealing with contradictory communication. This is then material for inquiry and dialogue between the coach and the coachee and rich material for relational learning.

Attention to language and communication

These levels of communication are interwoven in our language so that we will often experience both levels in dialogue. For example, much of our language has a bodily resonance so that we respond both cognitively and emotionally to what is said. For example, 'I feel as if I am doing well enough but I am not quite there yet', which brings to mind and body the sense of a tough journey. Or, 'I felt slapped by that negative comment from the CEO', which is a powerful communication at both levels! What the Boston Change Process Study Group (2008) makes clear is that we are dealing with interwoven strands of communication – the verbal content and the implicit, somatic and embodied. Working with an appreciation of this can support clients to be open to, and reflect on, the different levels of communication that they experience in their interactions both with the coach and with others in the organisation.

Clients often make use of coaching to explore difficult and challenging relationships they have with colleagues with whom they need to engage more effectively if they and their organisations are to be successful. How they respond to others and make sense from these interactions will be informed by their own relational templates and how they then make sense of their interactions based on explicit verbal content as well as what they experience and perceive at the implicit level. Many organisations still operate with rationalist ideas of communication as a process of logical transmission of universally understandable ideas. In reality interactions are often multi-layered, incongruent, what is said is not always what is meant, changes over time, and what is done does not always align with publicly declared intent (Armstrong, 2005; Schwartz, 1990; Vansina and Vansina-Cobbaert, 2008). Incongruence often arises because of a split between the public and private discourses in organisational life. The former 'official system' often rooted in ideals of organisational rationality, and the latter 'unofficial system' coloured and shaped by the emotions and subjectivities of organisation participants, which operate under the surface of what can be publicly acknowledged and thought about (Day, 2012). Helping clients to make sense of their own incongruence, that of their colleagues and what this might have to say about meanings, anxieties and assumptions operating under the surface of interactions can support greater connection, understanding and learning. It also allows for experimentation with new and more generative forms of communication informed by greater awareness of relationship dynamics, undercurrents and their meaning.

Meeting relational needs in the context of the coaching relationship

A relational orientation to coaching acknowledges and appreciates the basic human need for relationship, connection and support that is often denied and treated with suspicion in the individualist paradigm. We find it helpful to draw on Kohut's (1984) perspective of using another person as a 'self-object' to confirm our experience of our sense of self through 'seeing ourselves' in the eyes of the other (Kohut, 1984). In the highly pressured, technology-reliant contexts in which many clients work, individuals can experience isolation and disconnection from one another, transacting cognitively rather than relating in a more fully human-to-human way. Given the relational nature of the self as set out in Chapter 2, the quality of relationship with others is fundamental in determining the quality of relationship to self, how clients experience themselves, their resources, think and act. Relationally oriented coaching can provide a context in which coachees can experience being met and seen more fully, where more of their experience is witnessed and validated and their connection to *themselves*, their resources and creativity restored in the *meeting* with the coach. Over the years we have coached a number of senior HR leadership teams involved in driving significant operational change in their organisations. We have noticed that their experience of themselves as being creative, reflective and responsive becomes more and more contracted the more they focus primarily on driving change in transactional ways. It is necessary, particularly where problems and difficulties arise, to create contexts where they can meet, slow down and reflect in order to reconnect with individual and collective capacities for creative problem solving.

Kohut (1984) identified three areas of relational needs: the need for mirroring – being seen for who I am and having this reflected back to me; the need for idealising – the need to hold the other as someone to be admired; and the twinship need – the need to feel a sense of belonging, that there are others in the world who share my experience. Wolf (1988) later added the adversarial need, the need to engage in confrontation with a resilient other. These are referred to as 'self-object' or relational needs and continue to be important throughout our lives, especially at times when we may feel stressed or undermined and are in need of the support of another to affirm our self concept (see previous example). As coaches we have a golden opportunity to be there for our clients to reflect back what we see and feel of their experience (mirroring) and so support the integrity of their sense of self. We can restore a client's self-acceptance through communicating our own acceptance of them as they are, as well as appreciation for qualities we see that they may not yet see in themselves. If we have relational range as practitioners we will equally not shy away from confrontation, and may even allow ourselves to be idealised (briefly!). This latter experience can be important for coachees to feel they are in the hands of someone they can admire and can trust. This strengthens the relationship and offers the opportunity for coachees ultimately to access the very qualities in themselves that they see in the coach. We cannot recognise qualities in others if we do not have them at least in embryonic form in ourselves. As coaches we can also provide our coachees with a sense that we are a kindred spirit who understands what it is to face human dilemmas so characteristic of today's organisational environments. We can communicate that, given the challenges and complexities the coachee is facing, who wouldn't feel disoriented and confused! Connecting the client's experience to a wider context and communicating an empathic appreciation that the coachee's dilemmas and challenges (experienced at the individual level) are a function of both her own internal world and the wider context dynamics in which she is located and works, can supply a reparative dimension in the relationship in the course of authentic dialogue. This stands to reduce the isolation and loneliness so often experienced by individuals in the grip of individualist assumptions about needing to be superhuman, omniscient, self-sufficient, heroic and self-sacrificing.

Expanding range – the creation of new narratives to promote contact with self and other

Existential perspectives (Spinelli, 2005; Van Deurzen and Hannaway, 2012) stress that we are 'meaning-making beings' in that 'our unique form of evolutionarily derived consciousness has as its primary function the construction of a meaningful reality' (Spinelli, 2007, p. 26). Yet we are frequently faced with what may be uncertain and unknown, which may appear meaningless and so lead us to construct meaning from a rigid standpoint. These stances can then become inflexible 'truths', which we will adhere to even in the face of contradictory evidence (Spinelli, 2010). A central focus in the existential approach is to support people to tolerate uncertainty so as not to prematurely shut down on their experience in the interests of managing their anxiety in the face of meaninglessness, as in the case of rushing prematurely to action or a solution that is not thought through and considered. This is where coaches can have a valuable part to play in enabling clients to convert neurotic anxiety (predicated on a fear of loss of control) into a capacity to bear existential anxiety in the face of having to make meaning, choices and live with the consequences of those choices, and where outcomes cannot be guaranteed in advance. This can involve a number of components including the coach's ability to befriend her own anxiety; support the coachee to regulate affect and arousal; make use of mindfulness practices; pay attention to relationship dynamics and the meaning making process itself in the here and now, and be less focused on pursuing an ideal of the 'right answer'. Instead, development and the emergence of action strategies can be reframed as being no more than taking the 'the next step'. Coaching can enable coachees to review their narratives about themselves, their work, their abilities and their relationships in a contained environment where it is safe to explore, and where they will be supportively held in their anxiety while facing new perspectives on life and work. This is particularly relevant in the context of vertical development (Kegan, 2009; O'Fallon, 2012) where clients are letting go of attachment to familiar mental models and opening to broader and more complex perspectives on meaning making and reality which is inevitably unsettling.

Cozolino (2010) talks of the 'integrative' properties of language, since recalling a story requires the convergence of multisensory capacities across the left and right brain hemispheres, so that language integrates, organises and regulates the brain. For this reason we can see that creating meaningful narratives that cast new light on our experience, so that we do not need to shut down on our thoughts, our emotions or our sensory responses, performs a liberating function for the coachee and facilitates integration of self-experience. For Cozolino (2010) the evolution of the brain and the development of narratives have gone hand in hand. He sees narratives as serving a range of important functions which support us to think sequentially, provide us with maps for emotion, behaviour and identity and contribute to self-definition. Lived stories will allow us to integrate feelings, sensations, behaviours and imagery in conscious awareness and facilitate neural integration, so avoiding overwhelm such as dissociative responses where the client's capacity to go on thinking under stressful conditions shuts down.

This research supports the focus in relational coaching on creating an environment where coachees can identify disjunctions in their experience as they relive, in their interactions with the coach and others, earlier defensive (protective) patterns of relating and viewing the world. These have their origins in outdated organising principles that may have served them in the past but no longer support their growth, professional development and effective performance. This can be a challenging process as we inevitably feel anxiety and discomfort when we bring into awareness parts of our experience that we have excluded in the interests of survival, minimising anxiety and protecting relationships with others who have been important to us. These aspects may be revived and modified through the creation of a new narrative that includes these forgotten parts of ourselves, often related to using abilities or expressing needs that we excluded in the past.

A client may have developed a style of self-sufficiency in the face of early experiences where others were not forthcoming in offering support, believing, out of awareness, that having needs is pointless, 'I have to do it all by myself'. This pattern of interaction and the out of awareness beliefs which underpin it translate in the work context into an inability to delegate and make room for prioritising time for strategic thinking, networking and relationship building, which the client recognises is key to succeeding in a new role and progressing in the organisation. Unless this client can be supported to surface and rework the meanings and narratives he has constructed in relation to believing he has to do it all, having needs himself and seeking the help of others, he is unlikely to succeed.

Perls *et al.* (1951) used the term creating a 'safe emergency' for the client, in which the coach (in our instance) provides a balance of support and confrontation so that the person can experiment and try out new behaviours, new ways of construing their reality, and re-own parts of their sensory, bodily experience which they have shut down in the interests of survival. Bromberg (2011) talks of the importance of creating a space that is 'safe but not too safe' so that the client experiences the practitioner's ongoing concern for his emotional safety as well as a commitment to the value of the inevitably unsettling process of revisiting aspects of his past, where necessary, and always in negotiation with the client.

There is an argument, particularly in the solutions focused coaching literature, suggesting that any focus on the past is exclusively the preserve of psychotherapy and has no place in coaching, which should only focus on the future and strategising for success and change (Greene and Grant, 2006; O'Connell, Palmer and Williams, 2012). We are not proposing here that coaches should intentionally direct awareness to the past if not relevant. However, where clients make connections to familiar organising principles and can see their origins, and where this has direct bearing on their organisational role, performance and situation, it is important that coaches can respond sensitively and in ways that support learning.

Relationships at work do have the capacity to evoke relational templates, which have their origins in patterns of interaction formed in the past. This is particularly the case in superior subordinate relationships with their power to evoke early parent-child patterns (Krantz, 1993). The Ego States model in Transactional Analysis (Berne, 1961/1968) is primarily concerned with states of thinking, feeling and acting forged in the past and enacted in the present, and these perspectives have been gaining currency in organisational life (Hay, 2007; Sills, 2012, Newton and Napper, 2010). More recently, Popovic and Jinks (2013) have proposed a model of coaching that can integrate working at greater emotional and psychological depth and this resonates with a need we see to bring more range to coaching conversations for responding to a greater range of challenging development issues and contexts.

A client may re-experience the pain of his having had a very critical parent in the context of an appraisal conversation in which he is given much development feedback. In bringing his discomfort with the feedback process to coaching, he may be confronted with the fact that his strategies of driving himself hard and always striving to be the best cannot protect him from the vulnerability he still feels in the face of feedback that suggests he is less than perfect. In his striving to please others in order to stave off imagined potential criticism, he may have disconnected from an ability to reflect on and simply enjoy what interests him about his work and his situation. He may discover that what he has rarely permitted himself is the time to pause, take stock and reflect on his experience and that of others with whom he has to interact and collaborate. He may come to discover that by doing this he actually begins to think and act in ways suited to his role and the feedback he received, and find more meaning and enjoyment in what he does.

This example points to the need for coachees to re-connect with and re-own those aspects of their experience that they have excluded from their current narrative (to their own loss).

A female coachee left the country of her birth with her family at a very young age and, in order to ensure integration in a new country, was forced to switch languages and was instructed not to speak her first language any more. She did this very successfully at school and focused on the sciences. Subsequently, as an adult, she embarked on a business career. Then in her current workplace in her new team there was a man whom she realised spoke her first language and she spontaneously addressed him in this. They had a warm encounter, but what stood out for her after this was how she had cut off from her younger self at age five, including her creative interests, her spontaneity, and the ease of communication she felt as she spoke her first language. She had become very formal and intellectual in her approach to work and relationships, a characteristic that had led her boss to recommend coaching for her to develop her 'emotional intelligence'! Her chance encounter reactivated her past and she was able in her coaching sessions to re-integrate this early part of herself and the experiences associated with it. In the 'safe but not too safe' space of coaching she was able to deconstruct the narrative of her past and create a new narrative in which she reclaimed the fullness of her early experience, her warmth and playfulness, and integrated this into her adult life and professional role, resulting in improved relationships, greater engagement and collaboration among her team members.

The deconstruction and reconstruction of narratives that provide meaning for our experience and allow us to reclaim aspects of ourselves that have been 'lost to us' allows for fuller neural integration which supports a more secure, integrated sense of self. Creative growth and the successful realisation of objectives in coaching is linked to creating new coherent and integrated narratives that incorporate a range of aspects of ourselves that we may have ignored or associated with shame. These will then be stored in our autobiographical memory where we will be able to access and update our narratives as we grow and change and move into new areas of experience. In this way clients can be supported to develop the self-other awareness so vital for responding and acting into the complex system dynamics of today's organisations.

The creation of a 'third' reflective space to facilitate learning and change

The coach and the coachee can be thought of as creating between them a third reflective space from which they can both observe their interactions, their individual responses, their process of mutual interaction and the impact their individual behaviour has on the other. This process of reflection allows for the development of a meta-perspective on relationships and provides the opportunity for exploring the impact that each has on the other within an agreed contractual relationship.

The concept of 'thirdness' has been much written about in the relational psychoanalytic field.

Jessica Benjamin (2012) points out that a shared third is experienced as a cooperative endeavour. The two people involved in the helping relationship create 'a shared third as a vehicle of mutual understanding' (p. 109). This corresponds with the co-created relational space we describe in Chapter 5 . In their encounters both partners take responsibility for their contribution to the co-created process and reflect honestly about their own part in this. This requires a degree of courage and a willingness to confront their own contribution on the part of both the coach and the coachee. Essentially this involves a shared sense of responsibility for the relational process and a capacity to take the subtleties of this process seriously as data regarding the nature of what is emerging in the relationship field and what it might have to offer for learning and change to occur. It calls for an openness in the coach to address his own mistakes and blind spots, and reflect on how he may have impacted the coachee in a way that he may not have intended. Benjamin sees this as 'the creation of a space for recognizing and negotiating difference' (p. 124).

Winnicott's concept of a 'play space' in which learning and experimentation can take place is also useful here. Although he is talking about the psychoanalytic process, we consider that his ideas are equally applicable to relational coaching, especially where new meaning needs to be made in order to adjust creatively to complex situations and challenges. Effective coaching, like effective psycho-analysis 'takes place in the overlap of two areas of playing' (Winnicott, 1971, p. 38) that of the coachee and that of the coach. Both participants are aware that such a 'play space' is both 'unreal' and 'real' in the sense that we know that we are 'experimenting' in the coaching session with meaning making and action possibilities, and yet the learning that takes place may impact us profoundly at every level and open up new horizons for us beyond the coaching room in both professional and personal domains. There is a freedom in this type of experimenting or 'play' because we can explore a range of behavioural, emotional and cognitive options and then decide on reflection which of these we feel congruent with and can creatively and realistically carry into the world outside. This contributes to an effective use of the learning space in coaching and an opportunity to 'live' new options. As Winnicott (1971) says '. . . playing is an experience, always a creative experience, and it is an experience in the space-time continuum, a basic form of living' (p. 50). Panksepp and Biven (2012) report that all mammals share a 'play system'. They describe the functions of play as learning various competitive and noncompetitive social skills that promote the ability to communicate and facilitate social bonding. This seems to us particularly relevant in the context of a relational orientation to coaching and the need many clients present with to improve and influence working relationships in order to be successful in their enterprise.

The implications of this for coaches is that we need to be able to be open to the direct experience of being with our clients, allow whatever is emerging to make itself known. It requires a spacious orientation that does not presume to know in advance what might be relevant, but trusts in a process of collaborative meaning making or 'bricolage' as described in Chapter 5.

A newly promoted client in a challenging leadership role mentioned to his coach that ever since starting in the new job he had been having a vivid dream. Before he could talk about the dream his coach clearly indicated that she did not 'work' with dreams as she considered this more the territory of psychotherapy. The client persisted in referring to the dream and became flat and withdrawn every time the coach brought his attention to the contract they had to work on leadership. Given the client's persistence, his increasingly flat energy and disinvestment from the leadership coaching, the coach brought the situation to her supervisor. In the play space of the supervisory relationship she was able to acknowledge her own anxiety about potentially entering a different territory of exploration to that which she had imagined. She also saw that she was casting herself in the role of expert and assumed that she would need to analyse and make meaning from the dream, neither of which she felt skilled to do. With the support of her supervisor, she was able to expand her perspective to include the possibility of at least hearing more about the dream in order to discover what it might have to say about the client and the work, without having to know, in advance, how to make sense of it. The next time she saw the client, she felt more supported, spacious in herself and curious to know more. She said to the client that she might have been a bit hasty in deciding that the dream was not something that may be relevant, as it clearly was relevant to the client and, although she was not experienced in working with dreams, perhaps she and he could explore a little to see what potential relevance it might have. At this the client relaxed and told her that in the dream he was standing behind a theatre curtain about to perform in a play. The curtain opens and the audience erupts into peals of laughter and he experiences people laughing at him. He feels terribly ashamed and anxious, freezes and cannot speak his lines. It is at this point that he wakes up. Again, with her supervisor's words ringing in her ears, the coach resisted the temptation to interpret the symbolism of the dream from a position of authority and, instead, opened up to feeling with the client the experience of standing on the stage with hundreds of people looking and laughing at him. She found herself wondering what this might be saying about the client's experience of being in his new leadership role. She shared this with the client who became very animated and spoke for the first time of feeling out of depth, under immense scrutiny and doubting of his ability to carry it off. This opened up a fruitful conversation with his coach who was able to help him to normalise his disorientation and together they were able to focus on developing the internal support and connection with others to manage his anxiety in the face of the unknown. Through making space for more of the client's experience to be included in the coaching conversation, the coachee was able to examine the ways in which he was experiencing the transition into the new role and identify strategies for managing his challenges. He began to focus less on being the 'image' he had of how a leader should be (acting a part!), and was able to make more room in himself to discover what type of leader he could realistically become, given the demands of the role and the capabilities he had to draw on and develop further.

Benjamin (2004) points out that when we lose this sense of a third reflective space under stress or tension we revert to a 'doer and done to' relational dynamic where each person may see the other as at fault and not understand her/his own part in this co-created dynamic. At that point the possibility of negotiation and ownership of responsibility is frequently lost in the interests of being right! In this respect the development and maintenance of the third reflective 'play' space lies at the heart of effective coaching. When we lose that space and revert to a dyadic perspective, then we lose our perspective on the uniqueness of the other and that person's inalienable right to be different from us. Organisational demands, coach anxiety about reputation and getting results, can all exert pressure, making it difficult to protect the learning space. We consider it a responsibility of the coach to be sensitive to occasions in the dialogue when the reflective space is lost and to engage his reflective process in the interests of restoring this learning space.

Working with enactments and coaching alliance ruptures

Enactments occur when the coach and coachee interlock in a process, outside of conscious awareness that leads to discomfort, a sense of something not being quite clear, of avoidance of something. This is a significant departure from a more individualist/rationalist orientation to coaching where the coach is seen to act upon the client to bring about change through the application of protocols.

Typical enactments include:

- The coach becomes anxious about getting a result and reacts to the coachee's apparent lack of urgency or results orientation.
- Initially the coachee hangs on the coach's every word and the coach steps into an expert role, talking at length and offering multiple options, strategies and solutions, the coachee becomes more and more passive.
- The coach believes that the client could achieve so much more if only he were able to reflect on his feelings and so puts pressure on the client to talk about emotions, the client retreats further into his preference for thinking and logic.

Each person will tend to see their behaviour as the consequence of the other's behaviour (McLaughlin, 1991). McLaughlin takes the view that enactments involve shared behaviours and are located in an intersubjective field. Our tendency is to 'blame' the other and we are often reluctant to see our own part in the process: 'This coachee is just so resistant to any help that I wonder what I am doing here!' or 'This coach is a one trick pony, they don't get me or my situation'. Chused (2003) points out that enactments occur when one person's behaviour stimulates an unconscious conflict in that of the other 'leading to an interaction that has unconscious meaning for both' (p. 678). In the example above the coach's anxiety in the face of her own growing edge resulted in her closing off to considering the potential relevance of talking about a dream for her client and in so doing initially contributed to shutting her client down. Chused (2003) does not consider the enactment itself as necessarily helpful, its usefulness is that it points to aspects of the client's (or coach's) experience that he is not yet able to talk to or explore. We consider it vital in a coaching relationship for the coach to be able to initiate reflection on the nuances of the interaction and open to exploring his own and the other's emotional, sensory and body responses. This stands to bring more of the underlying assumptions that coach and client are working from into conscious awareness so that they can be considered. They may offer up information about the coach, the coachee, the relationship and the wider context. They allow coach and coachee to make course corrections where the coach might have failed to understand something important to the coachee. In this they provide an opportunity to consider the quality of the coaching relationship and the uses the coachee is able to put the conversation to.

A coach in supervision reports that with one of her clients she is feeling stuck and finds herself uncharacteristically having a host of judgements about the client who she experiences as having great expectations for the coaching, casting the coach as someone who has wisdom to bestow. In spite of being clear that she sees coaching as a collaborative enterprise she finds herself doubting her own ability and catches herself aspiring to an ideal (which she believes she is failing to live up to) of a capable and experienced coach who would not be feeling so conflicted and confused. She tells her supervisor she is even considering pulling out of the engagement. As she recounts more of her experience it appears that the client, as she portrays him, is also prone to judgements, fixed beliefs and harsh criticism of others. She catches that her self-doubt has been activated by experiencing a client who she fears could be highly critical of her if she does not 'deliver' what it is he thinks he wants, and which may or may not be what the coach has to offer. The coach goes on to say that she found herself reading back through the coaching literature to try and find a way forward, reaching for the authority of 'texts' from a place of heightened anxiety and lack of trust in her own ability to work things out with the coachee. As the supervision unfolds, she is able to gain a wider perspective and generate tentative hypotheses on the factors contributing to her felt sense of stuckness and concern. The organisation in which the client is working is highly competitive and critical, and the client faces a series of leadership challenges related to making a series of unpopular structural and operational changes. She notices that her own reaching for an answer to her stuckness mirrors the coachee looking to her to be the 'answer' to his problems. With her supervisor she begins to consider that she might be caught in an enactment but that the experience also offers an opportunity to sense into the range of factors giving rise to the situation she finds herself in with the coachee and what this might also be saying about him and the direction of the work. She reports in the supervision feeling less anxious and more able to reflect on the situation and wonders if this may also be what is needed for the client.

In her next session she shares with the client some of her reflections from supervision. He is able to name his anxiety and the fact that he is looking to the coach to provide expert knowledge. The coachee is able to say that she is very happy to offer perspectives from her long career as an OD practitioner if the client wishes this, and only he can choose how to make use of any learning. She is also able to own and disclose that, under pressure from the system and the client's expectation, she had found herself anxious and doubting of herself, but had reminded herself in supervision that it was not her job to provide the answers but support him to find his own way forward. This seemed to allow the client to talk more about how he was experiencing the challenges and the pressure he felt there was to achieve extraordinary results quickly in a complex and uncertain context. The coach experienced herself as being able to relax her pursuit of solutions, slow down her judgements and meaning making which, in turn, allowed the client to begin to manage his anxiety and identify priorities and action strategies for himself.

Peter Bluckert (2006) has devised a series of pointers to assess the coachability of different clients and who is most or least likely to benefit. He makes important points regarding the need for an absence of severe mental illness, considering coaching as inappropriate for anyone who is mentally ill. He then grades potential clients as having poor, average, good or excellent levels of coachability depending on a host of factors such as the extent to which they are experiencing inter-personal problems, how others perceive them, the degree of threat to their careers, quality of performance and motivation. Frameworks such as these are important in enabling coaches and sponsors to begin to assess suitability and imagined return on investment. Yet, they can also imply a degree of scientific precision where judgements are made about people ahead of entering into a relationship where, from a relational and social constructionist perspective, coach and coachee actually can never fully know what might in reality be possible for each client with a particular coach in their context.

Coaches and clients are also vulnerable to internalising ideals about performance excellence, which, while an understandable aspiration, can also fuel anxieties about being 'good enough' in the face of multiple challenges and complexities. The challenges of the VUCA world mean that many clients will experience at different times a range of interpersonal challenges, fear of career derailment, performance anxieties and difficulties in bearing confusion and uncertainty in the face of complex systemic challenges. It is also possible that motivation for coaching will at times be high, at others low or non existent for the same client. Attending to the dynamics of the coaching relationship, particularly enactments, allows coaches and clients to bracket the pursuit of ideals and be open to considering more of the complexity of the total situation they find themselves in and its effect on self experience, reflection, creativity and action.

The coaching relationship can become a vehicle for reflection on any enactment and so lead to new behavioural options. It is the exploration of the enactment, not the enactment itself that is transformative.

We have found the following questions useful:

- What is not being acknowledged here?
- What am I avoiding?
- What am I not seeing?
- What needs to be said here?
- What can I learn from my bodily response to this person about what I need to reflect upon?
- By thinking and acting in this particular way, what might I be missing that could be useful to me and the coachee?
- What might my experience be telling me about me, my client and the context in which we are working?

Aron (2003) offers some useful guidance to the professional helper to enable her to recognise when she has moved into an enactment. He points out that when we are engaged in an enactment, observation and participation are split apart. This means that the person either loses the ability to think or observe and gets caught up in an emotionally-laden interaction; or the person becomes detached, and too cerebral and analytic, and so quite out of touch with the other person (p. 628). We have found this observation of particular help in our work as coaches, supervisors and as trainers of coaches. Either of these polarities marks the loss of the reflective function, of the capacity to hold self and other in mind as interactive beings – the mentalisation function.

When enactments persist over time and are not addressed, they may lead to ruptures in the coaching alliance. A familiar enactment we often encounter in our supervisees is where the coachee seems unresponsive to the coaching or the coaching relationship and the coach finds himself working very hard to engage and interest the client, increasingly offering perspectives or suggesting exercises, all the while listening less to, and reflecting less on, his direct experience of the client in the present moment and what this might be saying about the out of awareness and unspoken experience of coach and coachee and the dynamics of the coaching relationship. By developing this reflective function and catching the enactment, coach and coachee stand to discover what might be wanting attention or be required for the coaching to take hold in a meaningful way for the coachee.

The importance of rupture and repair in strengthening the alliance

From the therapeutic literature and research, we recognise the importance of dealing with rupture and repair in relationships as a reparative process which leads to greater understanding and insight into one's own behaviour. Lachmann and Beebe (1996), drawing from research into child development, have extrapolated the importance of the process of addressing disturbances or ruptures and repairing these as equally important in adult relationships. We consider that this is also central to dynamics of the coaching relationship and the relationships coachees have with stakeholders and colleagues in their organisations.

In his early research Safran (1993) identified three characteristic styles of rupture that occur in a relationship: (1) the client misperceives or misunderstands the intention of the helping professional in a manner that is consistent with the client's core beliefs; (2) the client and the helping professional engage in a dysfunctional interactional pattern in which their core beliefs interlock, which reinforces the client's core beliefs; (3) the helping professional refrains from participating in such a characteristic pattern which may anger the client. Examples of these would be:

(1) If the coach invites the client to 'share his own ideas about the problem' and the client hears this as the coach being withholding and unwilling to share his own ideas with him.
(2) If the coach gets irritated with the client for not being open to engaging in the coaching and the client in turn gets angry with the coach for 'trying to force him into something against his will' and a battle ensues.
(3) When the client repeatedly asks the coach what she should do, then ignores the advice and blames the coach so that the coach then decides to 'hand the problem back to the client' to think about for himself.

Ruptures resulting from these types of interaction can lead to the breakdown of the coaching alliance. In subsequent research Safran, Muran and Samstag (1994) identified the behaviour in two main types of alliance ruptures: the client will either confront the helping professional in an attacking and dismissive manner with comments like: 'You're not helping me' or 'This is a stupid exercise'; or, perhaps more typically in coaching, may withdraw from the dialogue by shifting the topic, or rationalising, justifying his own behaviour or agreeing with the coach without elaboration or further comment. The conversational tone may feel as if coach and coachee are going through the motions, there will be an absence of a felt sense of connection and new meaning and insights will be thin on the ground. What is crucial is for the coach to be alert to these shifts in energy and communication, which he is likely to be aware of initially at a personal emotional and somatic level, and then, once he engages his reflective process, he will notice the corresponding nuances in the client's behaviour. De Haan (2008), synthesising the findings of his research into critical moments in coaching, comments that the critical moments outlined by coaches 'confirm that the key point in the coaching relationship that is challenging to them as coaches is when they arrive at that point of rupture in the coaching relationship, where there is anxiety or doubt on the part of the coach and/or client' (p. 148). He points out that these critical moments are potential opportunities 'for insight and change' (p.151), or, as we like to put it when teaching, 'not knowing is often a pre-cursor to discovery, stuckness a pre-cursor to movement'.

There is usually heightened emotion at such critical moments, which can lead to a creative repair of the rupture that opens up new areas for discussion, or it could lead to the ending of the coaching relationship. The more severe ruptures may involve serious violations of expectation and reinforce long standing self-protective beliefs, which will prevent onward movement (Gilbert and Orlans, 2011). However, we also wish to emphasise that the word 'rupture' is a very powerful term that suggests that something is sundered apart, whereas it can also refer to those instances when we 'miss' the coachee in our communication. Stern (1985) used the term 'misattunement' for times when we incorrectly identify the other's feeling state. Kohut (1977) used the term 'empathic failure' to describe the moments in which we are out of tune with the other. Noticing the nuances of these slight 'misses' in communication, changes in the felt sense of connection and exploring them with the coachee can be rewarding in terms of highlighting differences in relational style, learning that will be helpful in any organisational context. This can be a challenge to coaches who may be in the grip of a belief or assumption that they should somehow always know what the right thing to do or say might be and cannot tolerate their normal human limitations.

What is required of the coach at a point of rupture is the capacity to 'own his own part' in the process and to be open about his mistakes and misunderstandings, recognising that what he intended may not have been what was experienced by the other, or simply owning that at that point he 'lost it' and ceased to reflect, in the language of Transactional Analysis – that 'his Adult went on holiday'! The willingness to engage in exploring the co-created nature of the rupture will enable both participants to remain open to dialogue. For the coachee such an exploration may well be a new experience in that the coach is owning his part in the rupture, is willing to 'own his mistakes' and normal human limitations, and is there to facilitate the coachee to deal with what emerges from this process. This involves us in accepting differences in perspectives, while at the same time working toward restoring the connection between us.

Negotiating difference in the relationship

A relational orientation to coaching which privileges the intersubjective nature of human relationship and meaning making has implications for how coach and coachee acknowledge and work with inevitable differences between them. In fact, exploring and thinking together about differences lies at the heart of an effective coaching process. Benjamin (2012) points out that as relational thinkers we need constant accommodation and negotiation of different realities. The negotiation of overt or subtle differences in relating can be a challenge to both partners in the dialogue since it is often much more comfortable to revert to the position that my perspective is the 'right one'.

In the global economy in which we now live, coaches will often be coaching clients from different cultures, races, countries, religions, belief systems, class systems, organisational cultures to mention but a few possibilities (Cox, 2012). How do we and our clients negotiate differences that we may find hard to accept? How do we negotiate among the different constructions of reality we outlined in Chapter 5? How aware are we of cultural differences in how people approach problem solving or relationships with work colleagues?

What is crucial here is to develop an awareness of how even when people speak the same language, particular words will have a very different meaning and emotional resonance for people depending on their own particular histories. It is our task as coaches to be alert to this and attend to slight changes in voice tone or body language or gesture that may indicate that the other person does not 'feel understood'. Enquiring about what we observe and giving space to this exploration will often reveal that a significant emotional and cognitive switch has occurred in response to a word that we have used without realising its significance. An example is where a South African may say: 'Agh shame that sounds tough for you' in a sympathetic tone for them, which an English person may hear as criticism and as shaming them!

In the next chapter we shall explore further how differences can be a source of change and development.

Chapter 8

Relational integration

Implications for practice

> ... in a world of cause and effect everyone clamours to be a cause
>
> Gergen (2009, p. 51)

In the previous two chapters we have set out a number of perspectives on the micro dynamics of relational interaction and the ongoing co-creation of the coaching relationship. We have seen how a relational orientation involves paying close attention to sensing and thinking about the subtle, yet powerful processes that are experienced when two people come together in a coaching conversation in a particular context, and how these can be made use of in service of exploration, meaning making, learning and change. In this chapter we shall set out a number of practices of relevance to a relational orientation to coaching in order for coaches to consider how this might look and feel for the practitioner and coachee.

This is intentionally not a series of to do lists, protocols or skills divorced from any understanding of the underlying processes that give rise to them. Relational coaching is more of an orientation than a set of tools, although the orientation itself influences the ways in which particular skills and tools might emerge, be negotiated and experimented with. We assume that readers will be versed in the basics of coaching, and this chapter is intended to point to how practitioner orientation and practice might be expanded by integrating a more relational approach. This is a subjective and unique project for every individual coach involving sound theoretical underpinning, skill and personal development work on the part of the practitioner.

The perspectives that follow are in no way intended to be exhaustive. One of the distinct advantages of an integrative approach is that it remains open to discovering new relationships between theories and practice, and continuously researching collaboratively with clients and colleagues the validity and applicability of different approaches in different contexts.

Creating a container for the work – Paternal and maternal containment

For coaching to be effective there needs to be a container established for the work. Western (2012) sets out a model of containment which is particularly suited to coaching with a relational orientation, drawing as it does on relational processes experienced in infancy, and which are critical in facilitating learning and change in adult life. He sees coaching as a psycho-social process where our inner landscape (psycho) engages with and has to respond to the outer landscape (social). He identifies two types of containment. The first, paternal containment, is drawn from a Lacanian (2007) view of the father as a symbolic or metaphorical presence that represents the external world including 'action, activity, structure, form' (Western, 2012, p. 268), as well as complex relationships that have to be negotiated. It also includes an appreciation of difference and the reality principle – the fact of there being an external reality (as opposed to simply a closed individual inner world of feelings and thoughts), which has to be faced and negotiated. Paternal containment is important at both the start and the end of a whole coaching engagement as well as individual sessions. At the start of an engagement paternal containment is provided in the form of clear contracting and exploration of client and context expectations; clarity in relation to financial transactions, such as fees and cancellation policy; the number, duration, location and frequency of sessions and confidentiality agreements. It is also provided by ensuring that the physical location of the coaching is in a space conducive to the task, without interruption or distraction.

With maternal containment the metaphor of the mother represents 'the internal world, emotional containment, pairing and dyadic close relations, intimacy, oneness, harmony, play, creativity, thinking, formlessness and emergence' (p. 268). Based on the work of Melanie Klein (1959) maternal containment draws on the fact that the infant, lacking language and a capacity to make sense of experience in symbolic form such as words and mental constructs, projects feelings and anxieties that are experienced as overwhelming into the mother. The mother takes these projections in and, rather than reacting with her own emotion, panic or by ignoring them, is able to contain them emotionally. Maternal containment is the capacity to hold difficult emotions and responses and return them in a manageable form to the infant such as in an attuned and soothing response. Bion (1961) took up this idea in relation to group dynamics and also used it to inform his theory of thinking (Bion, 1962). Here he proposed that returned emotions were not only 'managed', but 'returned' in the form of meaning. In this way, raw emotions and direct experience can be converted into meaning and then thinking through the provision of maternal containment. This is central to enabling coachees to regulate their anxiety and make sense of their experience, think about their situation, their emotional responses and identify new strategies for action. It requires that coaches be sufficiently aware of themselves and practiced in managing their own anxiety and reactivity.

Maternal containment can provide a safe, trusting and intimate space in which to face personal and professional challenges, anxieties and complexities of the VUCA environment. It is the context in which coachees stand to feel supported and understood by their coach as seen in the previous chapters.

At the end of each session and engagement, Western (2012) stresses the need to reassert the paternal containment function in service of forwarding the coachee's action in the world. Balance is required between both maternal and paternal containment. Coaches under pressure to achieve quick results, busily rushing to technique, goals and solutions, risk missing the generative potential and opportunities for new associations and learning afforded by maternal containment. Similarly, without paternal containment towards the end of a coaching process, the coaching relationship risks remaining primarily a safe and supportive space, but one where changes in the external world are not made. At the end of a session, the coach needs to guide the client in identifying the implications of his insight for his action in the world along with strategies for making these a reality. In this way insight becomes transformation. Western (2012) stresses that maternal and paternal containment used in this way enable coaches to become freer, working with individual authenticity and creativity while also having a process that can hold and guide sessions. This is key in supporting coaches to bring more of themselves to the coaching process, which we shall explore in more detail later in this chapter, and enables a balance to be held between structure and space.

Integrating a phenomenological approach to collaborative inquiry and meaning making

A relational and integrative orientation to coaching privileges the subjectivities of coach and coachee. It is concerned with exploring how meaning emerges in the present moment context of the coaching conversation. As such, a phenomenological orientation to practice is particularly suited to working in this way.

Phenomenology is a branch of philosophy concerned with, among other things, whether reality is objective, external to our minds, or only subjective, created by our minds. It is closely related to existentialism and the study of how perception and meaning-making come about. Phenomenology points to a tension between objective and subjective forms of reality. While there may be an objective dimension to forms of reality, as in the atoms and sub-atomic dynamics that make up the paint, canvas and frame of a painting, the experience each of us has of the painting will be highly subjective and only exists in the moment of its perception. It can never be perceived in exactly the same way by the same person again. Each subjective moment of perceiving will be a unique experience in time (Spinelli, 2005).

These ideas are particularly suited to an orientation to coaching that is concerned with exploring how coaches and coachees make meaning together from their direct experience, rather than unconsciously mediating experience through existing knowledge, assumptions and protocols. This supports ongoing evaluation of whether the meaning that is being made is actually acting in service of a coachee's functioning in her specific context, her stated goals and context requirements. A phenomenological orientation also allows for an exploration of how the coachee is constructing his or her goals and what the underlying assumptions, processes and contextual factors might be that come to shape the structure and nature of coaching objectives. In Gestalt theory (Wollants, 2007; Yontef, 1993), and as we set out in Chapter 3, studying how meaning is made from experience and bringing this to awareness can, in and of itself, be a powerful catalyst for development and the construction of different meanings and perspectives, which in turn can lead to different action in the world.

Existential and phenomenological principles have given rise to a method for inquiring with clients into the nature and construction of their meanings and experience based on three practitioner orientations:

Principle 1 – The rule of epoché or 'bracketing'

The principle of epoché involves being prepared to put aside or 'bracket' whatever assumptions and presuppositions as coaches we might be bringing to a particular client or organisational context. It involves developing the capacity to pay attention to how our assumptions as coaches and familiar ways of making sense, and those of our coachees, inevitably mediate how we perceive and go on to act as a result. It requires of us that we open to multiplicities of meaning and relax attachments to any *one* way of seeing things. It is very easy in the world of coaching and organisational life to take a number of assumptions for granted. We might align with the perspective of a leader on their direct report who is to receive coaching and act as if that were truth. This would fix meaning in a particular way and inevitably colour and constrain meaning making going forward. Instead, from a phenomenological perspective, it would be very important here to be curious about how the leader's perceptions have come about and, if we are to practice bracketing, we would put these to one side in order to experience the coachee with a more open and spacious orientation. It is equally easy also to align unquestioningly with dominant organisational orthodoxies rather than inquire into them. Staemmler (1997) has coined the term 'cultivating uncertainty' to denote an attitude where practitioners actively work to hold any meanings they make lightly and tentatively, welcoming the possibility that what is understood is always partial and provisional. Meaning is seen to arise in a particular moment, and stands to change over time, in different contexts, and as more information becomes available. A phenomenological orientation requires coaches to become increasingly aware of, and be able to differentiate between, the experiential phenomena they encounter in themselves while being with their coachees, and the ways in which they infer from these experiences. As Gendlin 1962/1997) puts it:

Meaning is not only *about things* and it is not only a certain logical structure, but it also involves *felt* experiencing. Any concept, thing or behaviour is meaningful only as some noise, thing or event interacts with felt experiencing. Meanings are formed and had through interaction between experiencing and symbols or things

(p. 1., italics in original).

Principle 2 – The rule of description

At the heart of this principle is an invitation to the coach to describe what he or she sees rather than explain or interpret. This cuts across the tendency in all human encounters to rush to make meaning on the basis of pre-existing theories and models, which risk constraining the possibility for more data and new potential meanings and implications to emerge. We might notice that a client, who is talking about feeling frustrated by what he perceives as unnecessary control and bureaucracy in his organisation, every time he mentions his line manager begins to make a fist with his right hand. If we were to rush to make meaning we might decide (among a number of possible options) that this is a sign of aggression and possible hostility towards his line manager. If we were then to make an interpretation or frame a question along those lines (i.e. 'might you be feeling angry with your boss?'), we would be overly determining the client's experience based on our, non-negotiated, meaning making. Instead, following the principle of description, we would simply draw attention in neutral language to the phenomenon that has captured our interest by saying something like – 'I notice that whenever you mention your boss, your right hand begins to curl'. This enables the client to become aware of something that was hitherto out of his awareness. By noticing more of his feeling and embodied experience as he does this he is more likely to arrive at his own associations and meanings. In this case, the coachee identified that the curling movement and stroking the palm of his hand with his fingertips accompanied moments of mounting frustration. Rather than signaling aggression, it actually acted as a form of self-soothing and enabled him to regulate down his experience of mounting tension.

Principle 3 – The rule of horizontalisation or equalisation

As we study with our clients the nature of their experience and the meanings they are deriving from it using the principles of bracketing and description, this third principle invites us to resist ascribing any value or particular hierarchy of importance to the phenomena that we are exploring. We are encouraged to treat everything that emerges as having equal value or 'possible relevance' (Parlett, 1991). This allows more of the underlying meanings, motivations, contextual forces and coachee patterns to emerge and become available for exploration. Wollants (2007) refers to this as the 'total situation'. Surfacing more and more of the total situation in turn generates more and more potential options for experimentation and change. Aspects pertaining to the context or client's construction of reality, that had hitherto been out of awareness, now present themselves for consideration and, where necessary and desirable, for modification. By prematurely ascribing greater value to any one element, we risk constraining the possibility for novelty and new insights, as now meaning making will be mediated through what has been determined to be of value and often reinforced by taken for granted norms. The result is that other potentially equally relevant perspectives are likely to be dismissed as unimportant or missed altogether.

The phenomenological method is a useful orientation for coaches wishing to integrate relational principles into their practice as it supports the collaborative inquiry in action that is at the heart of this approach (Barber 2006a). It is consistent with maternal containment and supports cultivating greater openness to multiple meanings, which are always partial, contextual and changeable. This can be challenging at times in organisational contexts where clients and coaches can be under immense systemic and psychological pressure to have to make meaning fast and take quick and decisive action. At the same time, coaches who can integrate phenomenological principles into their practice can offer clients the opportunity to track more closely the ways in which they make sense from their experience and how often these meanings, if unexamined, can be the cause of unhelpful perceptions and resulting behaviours. This orientation is also particularly suited to transformational coaching and learning, as a phenomenological stance supports noticing and describing patterns, and enables underlying assumptions and action logics to be explored and expanded where desirable and necessary.

Integrating different forms of relating

John Nuttall (2012), drawing on the work of Petruska Clarkson (1995), outlines a series of relationship modalities that might arise in the coaching relationship and in relationships in organisational life – the working alliance, the transferential mode, the developmentally needed relationship, the person-to-person mode and the transpersonal mode. Each of these perspectives offers a way of understanding, identifying and reflecting on different dimensions of relating in the context of coaching and how they may be made use of by coach and coachee alike to facilitate learning.

The working alliance dimension points to paternal containment (Western, 2012), the relational and contractual bond the coach and coachee form in order to support the work. It brings into focus the importance of defining roles and boundaries and emphasises the need to, and possibility of, working collaboratively with others based on realistic expectations. We shall explore aspects of contracting in more depth in the next section.

The transferential mode of relating is drawn from psychoanalytic theory and refers to ways in which psychological experiences and relational templates from the past can be revived in the present moment and unconsciously shape perception, meaning making and behaviour. This is also the territory of enactments and interlocking organising principles outlined in the last chapter. Psychoanalytic organisational theory points to how organisational life can evoke material related to parent-child relationships, membership and survival anxiety (Czander, 1993; de Vries, 1980, 2006; Gould, Stapley and Stein, 2001; Hirschhorn, 1997; Menzies-Lyth, 1960; Western, 2013). This dimension enables coaches and coachees to understand how we can misconstrue relationships and interactions based on past experiences giving rise to dynamics detrimental to effective working in both the coaching relationship and encounters with key organisation stakeholders. These are particularly likely when anxiety is high in the face of complex personal, relational and organisational challenges.

The developmentally needed mode of relationship points to the intentional provision of a 'corrective, reparative or replenishing relationship or action' (Clarkson, 1995, p. 108 quoted in Nuttall, 2012). Originally recognised as a vital component in therapeutic change, it is now increasingly becoming recognised that attending to the relational needs of individuals is significant in leadership and wider organisational life where authentic concern for people is key to engagement, motivation and loyalty (Western, 2013). It is the territory of Kohut's (1977) self-object needs as outlined in the last chapter, and is central to coaches being able to participate in supporting clients to relate effectively to one another, access their inner resources and foster self-acceptance.

The person-to-person mode of relationship is characterised by the full acceptance of another's subjective experience, akin to Martin Buber's (1958) stance of I-thou. It is open to the experience of the here and now relational encounter. It involves opening to and allowing more genuineness and a fuller range of human experience than that prescribed by role identification, practitioner repertoires and social and cultural norms. It allows for the sharing of different beliefs, feelings, anxieties and vulnerabilities. It stands in marked contrast to playing a part, taking a fixed role or being what we think the other wants us to be in order to impress or keep ourselves safe. It involves an intimate encounter with self and other. In the coaching context it is what allows us to notice how we are being impacted by being with our different clients. While evoking anxiety in organisational environments where emotion and fuller human expression might be culturally constrained, it also serves to bring people closer together. This is particularly relevant where individuals and groups might be facing complex challenges and difficult decisions. It can evoke a sense of mutuality irrespective of hierarchy and a sense of sharing in experiencing dilemmas. It 'allows us to be human, with frailties and doubts, and yet still be valued, moderating the distortions of transference' (Nuttall, 2012, p.155).

The transpersonal mode of relationship is concerned with the more spiritual aspects of relationship. It draws on the esoteric, mystical, quantum and complexity perspectives, some of which we outlined in Chapter 5. It allows for the unexpected and apparently random to be considered as potentially relevant as in Western's (2012) Soul Guide discourse. It is the territory of values and intuition based action. For Clarkson (1995) it implies letting go of attachment to skills, knowledge, experience, preconceptions and even the desire to heal, or in the case of coaching to achieve a result or pre-determined outcome. It 'embraces spontaneity and imagination, and symbolises our ability to find meaning in what we do, allowing necessary disorganisation' (Nuttal, 2012, p. 155).

This is key in supporting more spaciousness in which new insights or 'aha' moments might arise through opening to a broader range of intelligence and knowing than that afforded by mental constructs alone and paying close attention to what is making itself felt in the moment.

Integrating greater use of self on the part of the coach

The term 'use of self' emerged in the context of relational perspectives in the world of psychotherapy (Rowan, 2002; Wosket, 1999) and entered the fields of organisational development and coaching (Rainey, Torbert and Hanafin, 2006). It refers to how in the context of an intersubjective orientation to development and growth the person, as well as the moment-by-moment experience of the practitioner, are considered to be a central instrument in the change process. In simple terms the coach brings to his or her work life experience, personality, professional development, particular training and orientations to coaching. In addition to this, the moment-by-moment experience the coach has in interactions with the coachee and their context also provides a rich source of information about the coach, the client, the quality of relationship between them, the context in which they are working and how this is permeating the field of the coaching relationship and intervention.

How the coach experiences him or herself in interactions with the coachee may offer up information about aspects of the client's relational style and patterning and may also point to more general ways in which the client impacts others as we saw in the previous two chapters. Here the coaching relationship can be thought of as being a 'fractal' or microcosm of the coachee's interactions outside of the coaching room.

This orientation requires that coaches be willing to sense into themselves more and track the physical sensations, emotions, thoughts, associations and images that arise in the context of being with a specific client in their context. It requires a capacity to hold both a sense of the direction of the work and a present moment focus, where what is emerging in the here and now is seen to always have potential bearing on the client's development of awareness and meaning making. In this way, coach and coachee are seen to be part of an 'embodied relational field' (Clemmens, 2012) where individual felt experience is seen as profoundly connected to the relationship, conversation and wider context in which the work is taking place. Cavanagh (2006) points to the importance of the body in the context of coaching where he says ' All conversations are embodied. All human communication is initiated in bodies, and is interpreted through bodies.

Our emotional states are the physical reaction we have to the communication in which we are involved' (p. 333).

Clemmens (2012) sets out four core skills and practices that are required for facilitators of change to attend to the embodied relational field and thereby make use of their own experience in service of the client. They are embodiment, attunement, resonance and articulation. Used together, these practices enable coaches to track in themselves and their clients the ways in which meaning arises from direct experience. It supports inquiry and meaning making to be grounded more in direct experience rather than abstract conceptualisation alone. It connects the visceral to the symbolic, the implicit to the explicit.

Embodiment

This is the experiential quality of the practitioner experiencing herself as a 'full self' as opposed to a 'role self' or 'pretending' in order to be seen as he/she would like to be seen (Yontef, 2007, p. 21). We can achieve this by becoming present to the breadth of our experience in the moment. Clemmens (2012) suggests we might notice our breath, feel our feet on the ground, notice the quality of our muscle tone in our bodies and faces, paying close attention to how we are orienting ourselves in relation to the client. These will be different in different contexts and with different clients moment by moment. He stresses that 'all of this process needs to be an ongoing discipline and as figural as my thoughts or theories about the client and our process' (p. 42).

This can represent a radical shift for many coaches who may be inclined to focus at purely the cognitive level of interaction asking questions and deploying techniques, processes and tools to elicit discovery and movement towards the client's originally stated goals. While this aspect undoubtedly has its place, embodiment is the first step to becoming more present to oneself in relation to an other and bringing more of oneself to the encounter. It can reveal felt dissonance between the coachee's stated goals at the explicit level and how he or she may actually feel and behave in relation to them.

Central to the practice of embodiment is presence, the coach's state and orientation to the coachee. Silsbee (2008) stresses 'your way of being is fundamental to your ability to produce genuine new shifts, insights and behaviours with those you coach. The coach is an instrument for the client's development' (p. 27). Nancy Kline (2013) points to the relationship between coach presence and the capacity for thought in the coachee – 'the quality of a person's attention determines the quality of other people's thinking' (p. 17). Fogel (2009) continues in this vein by discussing the value of 'slowing down and being in the subjective emotional present' (p. 23). Sills, Lapworth and Desmond (2012) describe presence as 'being in the here and now, ready to be alive to every facet of the moment' (p. 103). It is characterised by an aware sensing into oneself, being authentic, maintaining non-attachment to specific outcomes and attuning to the coachee and their context (Denham, 2006). It involves holding a tension between simply noticing experience and also being oriented towards a client's development and the relevance of what is arising for this objective. Denham-Vaughan and Chidiac (2007) describe this as 'fully being while doing' (p. 11). In this process the coach moves between 'grace' as a quality of receptivity to what is experienced and 'will' in the form of directed action or taking initiative in service of the coachee's learning and growth (Denham-Vaughan, 2005). This also mirrors the different qualities of maternal (grace) and paternal (will) containment. This form of presence includes the knowledge and information the coach brings to the relationship as a latent resource that may be called upon in different ways depending on what emerges between coach and coachee. The coach's objective is to be present and available to being impacted by the client moment by moment, and as responsive to the needs of the situation as she can be (Denham, Vaughan and Chidiac, 2007). It requires holding the tension of the polarities of receptivity and activity.

Attunement

Through cultivating a sense of embodied presence, which might also include preparatory activities in the coach such as mindfulness practices and body scanning, the coach is able to attune to the coachee. Attunement involves the opening or reaching out with our senses to whatever 'echoes' or shifts within us and our client. This requires the coach to be at least in part rooted in sensing into his felt experience while including the experience of the other in his awareness. We often teach students to practice sensing their bodies via a body scan with their eyes closed. Once they have connected with the feeling of their bodies we ask them to open their eyes and take in the sights around them while keeping 60 per cent of their attention focused on their sensations and only 40 per cent on the outside. Though initially challenging, this supports coaches to become focused on their body sensations as they are impacted by the coachee, and cuts across the tendency in many coaches to leave their connection with their bodies and focus their attention and energy in thinking. This is similar to tuning an instrument. If we take the idea of self as instrument seriously, then we need to practice increasing our sensitivity to being impacted at the levels of sensation and emotion as well as cognition. If a coach's attention is predominantly located in the realm of thought, listening to content, reflecting logically about what they are hearing, and scanning their memory of strategies and exercises, they will have less attention available for deeper listening and tracking of their own subtle responses. Attunement supports coaches to enter into a receptive mode and open to noticing what subtle and not so subtle shifts are occurring in coachees and in themselves. Clemmens (2012) stresses that in 'order to do this we must empty our task-oriented mind and allow our bodily experience to be part of the foreground' (p. 42). With attunement the goal is awareness of how the coach is being impacted by the client and also inviting the client to become curious about their sensory experience in relationship with the practitioner and context.

Resonance

Building on attunement, resonance is where we notice our own movements, breathing and posture in relation to the coachee, and stay present and open to what we notice as we are impacted at a bodily level. This 'staying with' allows what is emerging in us to become more developed and unfold. Clemmens compares this to being a bowl or resonant instrument (Clemmens and Bursztyn, 2003). This is an embodied form of empathy (Kepner, 2003) where we experience being touched and impacted by the coachee and where our own experience is shaped in this process.

Articulation

Articulation is the process whereby we allow that which is resonating to form into thought, language or gesture. Aspects of our sensory experience might unfold and amplify, they may then give rise to an image, thought or association, to a memory or theoretical perspective. It is the process whereby we put our experience into meaning through our own thought processes and then articulate this to our coachee in gestures, words and statements. Embodiment, attunement and resonance are closer to implicit modes of relating, whereas articulation moves into the explicit domain where experience is connected to language and thought. In earlier chapters we set out how change and transformation happen through the interplay of both implicit and explicit domains, and the four practices of embodiment, attunement, resonance and articulation allow coaches to move between these two domains whilst inviting their clients also to do so. This process corresponds to John Heron's (2002) hierarchical model of the human psyche where sensation and affect (feelings) give rise to the imaginal realm of experience, which includes the imagery of imagination, memory and perception. The next dimension is the conceptual domain of thought and language. Here our experience is translated into beliefs, assumptions and propositions about ourselves and the world. This domain is also mediated through existing guiding principles, assumptions, beliefs and theories. How these guiding principles arise or not is important to consider. Cavanagh (2006) describes how knowledge is an emergent property as opposed to something finite which is either acquired or lost, for example in forgetfulness. Access to knowledge moment by moment is 'shaped by our relationship to self and other – we can be rendered dumbstruck and lose our capacity to think in a particular conversation where we are being bombarded by questions' (p. 331). With this Cavanagh is commenting on the risk of those coaching approaches, which hold that the coachee has all the answers within him and that the coach needs to draw these out through questioning. A relational intersubjective orientation sees knowledge as arising where the subjectivities of coach and coachee interact and where differences can be explored and negotiated. In this way the coaching conversation is 'an organisation that emerges from the complex interaction of the coach and client – it is a co-created conversation'

(p. 337). This is also the territory of associative intelligence and 'bricolage', which we described in Chapter 5 , where new connections stand to be made by combining different realms of knowing and experience. In this co-creation, mental models and theoretical knowledge are re-membered (as in put together again), constructed, and emerge in the moment from 'within the complex responsive dialogue that goes on between people and within the person (p. 332).

When practicing articulation we listen deeply to the richness of data entering into the shared space between coach and coachee. We cannot help but notice and select certain aspects that capture our attention based on the filtering of our own experience, emotional responses and energetic attention. This is also the time to be paying attention to what might be missing, avoided or not being said, the practice Western (2012) refers to as 'minding the gap'. We pay attention to the feeling tone of what the client is saying and the feeling tone it elicits in us. Cavanagh (2006) describes how

> the client's communication enters into the coach's personal reflection space. Here it continues to interact with the coach's experience, mental models, emotions personality, history and so on, and we begin to see patterns as the client data elicits ideas, images, metaphors and theories. Meaning or knowledge begins to emerge for us in this process. This processing often continues post-session and during the coach's supervision.
>
> (p. 339)

'Articulation is the process of making known either to ourself or the client the embodied shifts current in the field as we sense them' (Clemmens, 2012, p. 43). The form, manner and timing of our articulation has to take into consideration the client's levels of resilience, maturity (including action logic for those coaches versed principles of vertical development), cultural and linguistic register, patterns of interaction, functioning, stage of the relationship and field conditions. The Gestalt principle of possible relevance (Parlett, 1991) is important here. All experience in the coaching relationship can be considered potentially relevant. This allows coaches and coachees alike to support an attitude of open curiosity, exploration and experimentation. Having said that, as coaches we also need to hold in mind aspects of the client's story, themes, context and stated goals when considering what to disclose or draw attention to. We track closely how implicit bodily experience and explicit cognitive processes are intertwined.

Integrating the ability to be a source of difference for the client

Much coaching theory has stressed the need for the coach to be a more neutral participant in the process, whose main focus needs to be on the client's experience, facilitating and evoking client insight in the form of skilled questioning. Understandable concern has been expressed over coaches offering advice from an assumed expert position, and this has resulted in a reductive and pervasive belief that sharing of one's direct experience and perspectives on a situation should always be off limits in a coach's practice repertoire.

From a relational, intersubjective perspective, coach and coachee differences are seen as a vital and necessary source of learning potential. Stacey (2000) has identified three factors that contribute to a free flowing and generative conversation – connectivity, referring to the need for rich and meaningful themes, what in Gestalt are referred to as figures of interest (Leary-Joyce, 2014); anxiety as an inevitable component when one is faced with the unknown and meanings that are emergent rather than pre-determined – too little anxiety and the conversation loses energy, too much, and anxiety shuts down thinking as was seen in earlier chapters; diversity which supplies necessary novelty for new meaning to emerge. Coach and coachee will hold different perspectives and it is these differences that provide essential levels of misunderstanding and cross-fertilisation needed to stimulate new connections and support the processes involved in bricolage as set out in Chapter 5.

Articulation of any difference needs to be offered in a spirit of collaborative inquiry. It is important here that as coaches we resist any pull to become attached to what we are noticing or the meanings that are emerging. There is a risk that our own anxieties about being seen to be clever, experts, insightful, value adding and successful can also get activated here and we can find ourselves prematurely wedded to a position. As with all interventions where we are articulating a sensation, perspective, memory, image or thought, the attitude of 'hinting' applies (Phillips, 1998). Hinting is an attitude or orientation not a practice. A hint can only ever be taken not given. If we think we can give a hint, we are inevitably caught in a linear and deterministic exercise of pressuring the client and pushing for a particular direction or outcome. Hinting works both ways. The coach, listening closely to the coachee might pick up on a particular use of language, notice what is not being said, sense incongruence between narrative content and the client's body process and emotions. These signs can be thought of as unconscious hints from the coachee as to how he is organising his experience and meaning making. In turn the coach articulates his response to what he is hearing which, equally, can only ever be a hint at some latent possibility that *only* the coachee can choose to pick up on or not.

This can be challenging to cultivate. Over the years we have seen many students and supervisees who are caught in assumptions about needing to demonstrate skill and value. Organisations in the grip of individualist and linear notions of change often require that we talk to the value we can offer and what we can do for the client and for the business. This is still a feature of many of the organisations we work in. With a relational orientation to coaching, the focus is not only on what the coach can do for the client but equally on what use the client might make of the coach's responses and thinking aloud. In this way insight, value, impact and outcome are not seen as being bound up primarily with the skills, capabilities, track record, level of accreditation and energy of the coach (which again risks coaching becoming an instrument of social manipulation and control), but as emerging out of the dynamics of relating between coach, coachee and context. Coaches need to track closely the impacts of their gestures and articulation with each client moment by moment. They need to remain alert to when a coachee might be overly compliant and quick to pick up everything a coach says, or, equally, when a coachee might appear overwhelmed, distracted or distant as a result of experiencing the coach's intervention as impinging on their own thought processes.

Cavanagh (2006) describes the freshness of this form of knowledge generation where coach and coachee can enter into a mutual and generative conversation fueled by the diversity of their individual subjectivities:

> The knowledge that is elicited is *new* knowledge – we coaches see it in the connections between what the client is experiencing and our own experience and understandings. When we are truly engaged in the conversation, this emergent knowledge has the character of insight, rather that the mechanical overlay of our preexisting models on the client's situation. It is an 'aha' experience (Lewin and Regine, 2001). Yet the insight is tentative until shared and agreed.
>
> (p. 339)

Any articulation or intervention on the part of the coach then, is an informed experiment, the offering of a possibility, to discover what use, if any, the client can make of it in their context and in service of their learning, knowledge generation and the broad parameters of the contract.

The coach's role is to contribute to creating conditions in which this might happen. Through articulation and sharing her perspectives, based on inner experiencing and reflection, the coach 'puts this transformed data back into the shared space for ongoing consideration . . . the coachee then picks it up and, all going well, takes it into the crucible of his own internal dialogue' (p. 339). The conversation continues in this way until coach and coachee have developed together enough shared understanding or shared mental model that opens up the possibility for new and differently informed action on the part of the coachee. This way of working is more in keeping with a post-modern orientation to coaching where assumptions about expertise and authority are less certain and taken for granted. Cavanagh (2006) also cautions against the coach becoming too identified with or wedded to a perspective – as might happen if the coach is overly identified with being an expert – 'when our theories and models move from being perspectives that nourish the conversation to the necessary conclusion of that conversation, they have moved from being information to ideology. When this happens, we as coaches have moved from a stance of curiosity and service to one of coercive arrogance' (p. 342). Or as one of our supervisors puts it 'it is very difficult to have a generative conversation with someone who knows what they are talking about!' (Wainwright, 2016).

Integrating broader perspectives for goal setting, assessment of change and articulation of value

Organisations are understandably concerned with the uses coaching is put to and the potential value it can bring to any business. Historically value has been determined on the basis of hard, demonstrable and behavioural outcomes in the coachee that can be seen to contribute in material ways to the organisation. This particular bias has its roots in the positivist and modernist traditions with their emphasis on predictability, control and efficiency (Cavanagh, 2013). At the same time, once we begin to consider coaching as an emergent process of collaborative meaning making, often in the face of increased complexity and uncertainty in human systems, it is necessary to broaden the ways in which goals are framed and value and impact might be assessed.

Complexity perspectives on human systems see goals, the outcomes of actions, as unpredictable, particularly as time frames extend forward (Stacey, 2003 cited in Cavanagh, 2013). There is an openness here to seeing goals as fluid and emergent. What may be articulated as a goal at the start of a coaching engagement provides focus and intention, but may also undergo refinement as the work unfolds and new perspectives emerge about a coachee's experience and the context in which he is working.

A relational and contextual orientation sees value not simply as determined on the basis of hard goals, tangible outputs and whether they have been achieved, but is also open to considering any other measures that may have relevance in a particular context at a particular time. Value is seen as also having subjective measures that co-emerge between all protagonists in the coach-coachee-context constellation. This broader orientation also accommodates the reality that change can happen at many different levels and that it can take longer than a coaching engagement to see the full impact of a particular coaching intervention.

Coaches integrating a more relational orientation in their practice have a role in educating clients and sensitising their organisations to a broader range of thinking about measurement. In addition to observable behavioural outcomes, equal importance might be given to the subjective reports of the coachee, relevant stakeholder feedback, the coach's own meaning making and perspectives. These might include beneficial shifts in energy and state of being, new knowledge and information, greater self confidence, greater clarity about growing edges, greater resilience, well-being and capacity to bear ambiguity and go on thinking on one's feet. All of these impacts are significant in enabling greater awareness and creativity required for navigating the complexities of organisational life on an ongoing basis. They support the development of 'perspective taking capacity', which Cavanagh (2013) describes as 'a person's capacity to understand, critically consider and integrate multiple competing perspectives into a more comprehensive perspective that enables adaptive action' (p. 168). In this way, in addition to whatever short-term objectives an individual may bring to coaching, coaching also stands to equip coachees with perspectives, reflection skills and awareness that continue to be of use long after a specific coaching engagement has ended.

From a Gestalt psychology perspective this capacity to reconcile and optimise the multiple tensions and complexities coachees face, internally and externally, into a meaningful resolution and timely action has a creative and aesthetic dimension to it (Mann, 2010). It is akin to the multiple pigments and brush strokes, light and shade of a painting being brought together into a finished picture. In terms of living an honourable life in good faith, the resolution must not be just driven by individual needs, but must also include authenticity and sensitivity to the wider contexts and impacts of individual actions on others (Crocker, 2004 cited in Mann, 2010).

It is a feature of organisations considered to be operating with greater capacity for navigating complexity that over-reliance on hierarchy and control mechanisms is relaxed in favour of enabling individuals, at all levels, to resolve creatively, in the form of aware, collaborative and experimental action, the challenges they face (Laloux, 2014).

Coaches opening to this expanded orientation to capturing and articulating value need to be constantly monitoring the uses the coachee is able to make of the coaching conversation and relationship with the coach. There is a need to be alert to the emergence of new information, the effects of this on initial goals and the flexibility to re-contract and incorporate this new knowledge into collaborative sense making.

In conclusion, the following basic considerations offer a way of thinking about the effectiveness of an intervention that is not predicated on meeting pre-determined and/or hard goals alone:

- That the coachee can make use of the coach's intervention (gesture, articulation, offer) in some way in service of meaning making and learning.
- That the intervention balances attention to the individual and the requirements of context, and supports self-directed and conscious resolution and responses in the coachee.
- That the intervention is executed by the coach with congruence and appropriate skill.
- That the intervention does not seek to impose the view of the coach, to harm or exploit the individual and their context.

Section 3

Applications

Chapter 9

Shame and vulnerability

The experiences that dare not speak their name

> ... forcing our natures to behave in a 'shouldistic' way is an attempt to actualise a self-image rather than the self
>
> Perls (1969)

In this section we turn our attention to a number of perspectives on coaching and organisational life that come into particular relief with a relational orientation to living and coaching practice. We begin with considering the nature and impact of shame, an experience which is profoundly interwoven with our human vulnerability and fundamental need for connection.

The experience of shame

Shame, and its milder form, embarrassment, are the feelings that can alert us to when we might have transgressed an acceptable range of behaviour in a particular context. As contexts vary, what is expected and accepted will change from place to place and situation to situation. Different individuals based on background and culture will also hold a range of beliefs and self imposed permissions and limits on how to be.

One of the useful functions of shame is to maintain norms and social cohesion, and yet it can also result in constraining expression, imagination and creativity if it becomes too potent a guiding force in an individual's life or organisation's culture. The experience of shame is closely bound up with the basic and fundamental human need for connection to others and anxiety in relation to whether we belong, are welcome, acceptable in others' eyes, or likely to be rejected. Brenne Brown's extensive research into shame has shown how we are hard wired for human connection (Brown, 2013; 2015). This makes us acutely sensitive to the possibility of disconnection whether we are conscious of this or not. She describes shame as 'the fear that something we have done or failed to do, an ideal that we've not lived up to, or a goal that we've not accomplished makes us unworthy of connection' (Brown, 2013, p. 68).

The direct experience of shame is characterised by feelings of exposure, self-consciousness, inner torment, judgement, comparison with others and often vicious self-criticism. We can feel totally exposed, giving rise to blushing and the wish that the ground would open and swallow us up. We experience a deep and profound sense of failure, lack, defeat, alienation, and a fundamental and pervasive sense of deficiency (Brown, 2013, 2015; Cavicchia, 2012; DeYoung, 2015; Kaufman, 1992; Orange, 2008). Unlike guilt, which can often be alleviated with a heartfelt apology, shame can be very difficult to work through given the depths to which we feel, in the grip of shame, fundamentally and irreparably flawed.

These vivid descriptions admittedly point to the more acute experiences of shame, but most of us and our coachees will have experienced moments of self-doubt, concern about how others might perceive us, or found ourselves comparing our attributes and achievements to those of others, wherein we end up feeling diminished, less able than we might actually be, less spontaneous and free, and disconnected from our own sense of capacity and worth.

Individualism and the denial of vulnerability

In earlier chapters we have set out how a relational orientation to coaching stands in marked contrast to the individualist paradigm. It is the very nature of the individualist paradigm that contributes to the arising of shame experiences and the difficulty in naming and exploring them, the antidote to which is a more inclusive and supportive relational orientation.

Of particular significance in the context of shame is the premise from within the individualist paradigm that any kind of vulnerability or dependency on others is fundamentally weak, infantile, inferior and effeminate (Lee and Wheeler, 1996; Wheeler, 2000). The assumption here is that everyone needs to be out for themselves, and so any form of vulnerability and need for connection is often tinged with suspicion. This gives rise to the fact that feeling shame, which inevitably points to this need for support, is often experienced as exposing and shameful in itself. As a result we develop a range of strategies for covering up our inevitable and ordinary human vulnerability. This results in further disconnection from others and the inability to reach out for support. Brenne Brown (2013) has shown that the emptiness and isolation that this breeds is often what underlies attempts at self soothing such as food, alcohol or drug addiction (whether illegal or prescribed). She cites statistics suggesting that currently Americans are more obese and more medicated as a nation that ever before (Brown, 2013).

The construction and celebration of disconnected self-reliance also has roots in archetypally masculine (Woodman, 1992) notions of health and functioning. Here growth, maturation and psychological well-being are predicated on an ever increasing capacity for autonomy and independence. From within this frame, any need for emotional support, or occasional dependence on others in order to go on feeling and functioning well, takes on alarming connotations of dis-ease and regression to unhealthy and infantile states of mind. Instead what is celebrated, and often financially rewarded in corporate life in the form of bonuses and other incentives, is heroic self-sufficient striving to achieve extraordinary feats and status for individuals and the organisations they serve. What are then discounted and disappeared from the public domain are the loneliness, addictions (including workaholism), failed relationships and cost to health and well-being that this striving can give rise to.

From a complexity perspective the opposite forces of connection (collaboration, community) and competition (separateness) (Lewin and Regine, 2000; Stacey, 2001) have to be worked with and held in a creative tension to avoid the extremes of each polarity if not tempered by the other. Yet it is the denial of human vulnerability that has its roots in the individualist paradigm, and suspicion of the need for human connection, that keeps many societies, organisations and clients oriented towards competition, individual agency and striving, denying them the balancing and creative potential of greater collaboration and relational support, which in turn contributes to a host of social and planetary ills (Eisenstein, 2011, 2013; Laloux, 2014).

The age of disconnection – Narcissism, self images and ego ideals

The individualist paradigm is also implicated in the construction of particular individual ideals and self images which become incorporated in enculturated meanings and expectations about what is considered to be required in order to be successful and happy in a particular context or society. It gives rise to an orientation which privileges the personality or ego, the images and ideas we construct about ourselves, identify with and which come to represent who we take ourselves to be, what we associate with success and what we aspire to.

Given how the human personality develops through the influence of others and the environment, it is also inevitable that many of us and our coachees can get caught in identifying more rigidly with certain self-images and striving to live up to those images which are also sanctioned by the society and organisations in which we live and work. Transpersonal and spiritual perspectives consider this identification and striving to be at the heart of the human ego and ego activity (Almaas, 1996a, 1996b). Through identification our sense of self becomes fused with these images and ego ideals and we experientially take them to be who we are. In this way we risk becoming in thrall to a virtual reality based on images rather than a deeper bodily connection to the richness and breadth of our human experiencing, our authentic desires, subtle body states, emotions and inevitable human vulnerabilities.

Identification with images drives a host of egoic striving activity. An image is a narrow representation in the mind of a reality. It is not directly connected to an authentic experience of reality in the moment. To the extent that we are in the grip of the misunderstanding that the image is what is real, we need to work hard to maintain it. The image acts as scaffolding, shoring up a holographic sense of identity. Without it we lose a sense of who we are which is experienced by the ego as extremely threatening. What is in fact a psychological threat can feel like a threat to existence itself. Our activity will be dictated by the particular images we are in thrall to. These include the accumulation of wealth, status and the acquisition of all that is associated with it from cars to houses, idealised body images, aspirational lifestyles, the achievement of intellectual prowess, fame and extraordinary accomplishment.

These aspirations undoubtedly can motivate some individuals to achieve great things, but can also be fixations which become ends in themselves, pursuits which disconnect individuals from deeper meaning, purpose and satisfaction given that they are driven by shoulds – what they have internalised as those aspirations that are implied to confer a sense of self esteem – rather than an authentic connection with what they might actually and authentically feel and desire.

Where self esteem and identity are overly fused with achievement and accumulation, individuals can become trapped in a permanent striving for the next bigger and better acquisition, promotion or experience, unable to derive pleasure and satisfaction from absorption in the present moment and a wider range of sources of satisfaction, meaning and purpose than simply the pursuit of ego ideals and images of happiness. Failure to live up to these ideals also causes shame as a feeling of being unworthy. As such, shame is also closely bound up with ego activity.

The striving to live up to ego ideals is closely policed by the 'superego'. The part of the personality first described by Freud (1911, 1923) as the 'uber Ich' in German, literally the 'above I', denoting the experience of an inner critic or judge that constantly evaluates our performance against the ego ideal and compares, criticises and judges us whenever we fall short. This can only, inevitably, be a frequent occurrence given that ideals, by their very nature, are rarely attainable. Where they are attained, enjoyment is usually short-lived as the superego has a way of finding yet another, or even greater ideal, to put in its place.

Yet who we can come to know ourselves to be is more than simply the images and ego ideals we hold about ourselves in our minds. From a relational, post-modern, perspective the self is seen to be a fluid process with vast potential for choice, meaning making, experimentation and creativity. Spiritual perspectives on the self (Almaas, 1996a, 1996b) also point to the importance of locating our sense of self more in the present moment flow of direct experience which, as a result of practices such as mindfulness and meditation, can come to be less unconsciously mediated through beliefs about self and the world, expectations formed in the past, and striving for an imagined future in which ego ideals and permanent happiness are attained. Rather, our own sense of who we are is more rooted in a connection to all of our felt experience, which includes our vulnerability as well as strengths. Mindfulness is increasingly gaining in popularity, offering as it does, practices which support dis-identification from mental content and images, and greater connection with a more direct experience of being (Kabat-Zinn, 2004).

Narcissism

The fixation on image and the discounting of deeper, painful experiences of emptiness and vulnerability are at the heart of the personality style of narcissism. We are not talking here of narcissism primarily in a pathological sense, but as the inevitable nature of the human condition whenever we are in thrall to an ego ideal or image, rather than connected to our direct experience as in the quotation from Fritz Perls at the start of this chapter.

Our fundamental human vulnerability to physical and emotional pain and need for authentic connection and security are denied in the pursuit of these individualistic ideals and shoring up of a 'false self' of images. Here others are related to primarily as objects to be manipulated in service of individual goals and in order to have reflected back the particular qualities an individual wishes and needs to be recognised for. The resulting isolation and profound emptiness act as a further spur towards more and more gratification and pursuit of idealised self-images. As many people will have experienced, these can never be sufficient or enduring given the denial and, therefore the lack of fulfillment, of the basic human need which underpins the behaviour – that for meaningful connection to oneself and to others.

The experience of shame, whether it is named as such, inevitably points to this often denied and defended against vulnerability and human need for connection. While many coachees may not have a conceptual or conscious understanding of shame, they can come to coaching with experiences which indicate they may be experiencing this phenomenon. These can include a preoccupation with self image and sensitivity (at times acute) to the perception of others (and particularly feedback) based on the need to have self images constantly shored up and reinforced by mirroring from others; exhaustion as a result of constant workaholic striving to be perfect; a lack of meaning and purpose in their personal and professional lives as a result of having disconnected from what they desire; the inability to set appropriate boundaries for fear of what others may think of them if they say no.

Developmentally, we are extremely vulnerable as children to taking in and believing negative perceptions of others such as parents and significant caregivers. This is related to our dependency on adults for our survival when we are young, resulting in being willing to believe the adult's version of us as bad or lacking. This willingness to introject (the term used in Gestalt to mean 'taking in without question') another's beliefs is based partly on the child's lack of capacity for discrimination given his age, and also serves to maintain a connection with a significant 'other' upon whom survival depends by submitting to their will and power, thereby reducing the risk of even greater disconnection.

Although this pattern is established in infancy, it can pervade adult life and fuels our sensitivity to the approval of others including managers, leaders and organisation peers. Furthermore, the understandable emphasis in many organisations on assessment, performance appraisal, individual and collective reputation, creates conditions in which the experience of shame is a very real potential. As a result, coaches and coachees can become externally oriented, extremely sensitive to what others think.

The respected Jungian analyst Marion Woodman, whose life has been dedicated to studying the human addiction to images, describes how, if we have come to depend primarily on the external approval of other, community or organisation to confer our sense of well being and nourishment, we remain 'starving' in relation to ourselves, disconnected from our own internally experienced, sense of identity, emotional life, well-being, desire, capacity for creativity and meaning making (Woodman, 1982).

There is an important distinction to be made here between what may be actual qualities of capability and competence, which an individual has and can draw upon, and the *image* of being competent and capable with which an individual is identified, and which is threatened every time life-experience and challenges call it, temporarily, into question. Nowhere is this more noticeable than in organisational life.

Ego and organisation ideals

In his seminal work *Narcissistic Process and Corporate Decay* Schwartz (1990) has shown that the individual tendencies we have to create our identities based on identification with self-images gives rise to a phenomenon whereby individual ego ideals become fused with the ideals of the organisation in which people work. This means that individuals, often out of conscious awareness, become very preoccupied with living up to the expectations the organisation places on them and its cultural norms, and also with maintaining the particular image the organisation wishes to promote to the world – the 'organisation ideal'. Brenne Brown terms this being hostage to pleasing, performing and perfecting (2013). Schwartz (1990) points out that this in part explains why whistleblowing is so difficult, even in the face of overwhelming evidence that an organisation is involved in dangerous, unethical or illegal behaviour. This can happen in spite of there being a host of factors which suggest the organisation is deviating in its practices, sometimes greatly, from the image it wishes to maintain. More often, this concern with belonging and aligning with the ideal (as image) can also make it difficult to question processes and practices which might be less than optimal, particularly where there is an investment at senior levels of an organisation in maintaining the status quo. Again Brenne Brown has described that where there is a marked gap between an organisation's espoused values (what it says it is about) and values in use (how things actually happen) then cynicism, alienation and disconnection are inevitable (2013).

The ideals of omnipotence and omniscience

Two particular products of the individualist paradigm which operate in organisations are the individual and organisational ideals of omnipotence and omniscience (Lapierre, 1993). Failure to live up to them can be a profound source of shame in clients and coaches alike.

Omnipotence refers to a set of beliefs, assumptions, images and feeling states associated with the ideal of being able to achieve anything one puts one's mind to and directs activities towards. Omniscience is a state of mind where we imagine and feel as if we know all we need to know in order to function in a particular context. It is a familiar ideal for those clients and coaches alike who are identified with being experts and needing to be right, needing always to know what should be done or said. This phenomenon is perfectly captured in the expression 'knowledge is power'. As ideals, these states of mind are grandiose and disconnected from the complexities of a social reality where knowledge and meanings are subjective, emergent, partial and provisional, and where certainty and predictability prove to be unreliable in light of the multitude of factors and variables that give rise to situations coaches and coachees find themselves in.

Nevertheless, these ideals can exert a powerful force in coaches, clients and the organisations they work in, where all can feel under enormous pressure to have to know, or be able to do, precisely what is required, and quickly achieve outcomes perceived to be desired. This is not to say that feeling committed and capable, or having expertise and deep knowledge in a subject area is not desirable or useful. The difficulty is that when ideals of omnipotence and omniscience are governing how people think, interact and take action, there is little room for multiple perspectives, partial understanding, intuition, subjectivities, uncertainty or complexity, and the discovery and creation of new knowledge and practice that is rooted in a deeper understanding of context. The pursuit of certainty dominates with no room for befriending the experiences of not knowing and vulnerability and developing the capacity for anxiety to be tolerated and thought about.

An example here might be a leader who engages subject matter experts in the grip of a grandiose idea of needing to be right, precise and certain, whereas what might actually be required by the context is agility, pragmatism, and a little calculated risk taking. The pursuit of meticulous detail may need to be relaxed in service of 'good enough' experimental action. When complex situations present themselves, where there is no obvious solution or immediate resolution, aspiring to ideals of omnipotence or omniscience (both forms of perfectionism) can make it difficult to slow down and explore the nature of the presenting problem, and the ways in which a client is perceiving and thinking, in order to create conditions where new knowledge and strategies might emerge and be co-created – a vital and necessary requirement of human organising in complex, uncertain and ambiguous times, and a process which lies at the heart of a relational orientation to coaching and consulting.

Instead, often, anxiety and shame in the face of not knowing drive people to rush into applying old knowledge to new problems in the hope of being able to solve them. Individuals may attempt to alleviate anxiety by rushing into activities, doing anything to reduce anxiety even if what is done is automatic, not thought out and even detrimental to people and their organisations. Some coachees and their organisations might experience paralysis and procrastination as a result of striving to predict outcomes and be certain about what may not actually ever be fully knowable in advance. Add to this the shame based anxiety related to how people view one another, and the scene is set for posturing, arguing, the taking and defending of positions. If a leader's sense of well-being is fused with needing to be 'right' there will be too much at stake to embrace uncertainty, risk inquiry, reflection, dialogue, collaborative meaning making and changing one's mind in light of new information.

Many of the complex situations leaders face are of the order of 'wicked problems' (Watkins and Wilber, 2015) where there are no obvious solutions and where resolution of some kind often creates a host of problematic unintended consequences. This can be very challenging to the assumptions embedded in the ego ideals of omnipotence and omniscience, of needing to be able to take fast, logical and effective action based on knowing or working out precisely what is needed. Here we see again the influence of the individualist paradigm and positivist traditions. Assumptions about linear causality, the existence of an objective reality that can be analysed, broken down into constituent parts and their workings understood, predicted and generalised, inform the ideals of omnipotence and omniscience. There are times when this might be appropriate and fit for purpose and context, such as in material precision engineering, yet the complexity, intersubjectivity, irrationality and human system dynamics of many organisations, along with market and political volatility, mean that there are often many challenges that do not lend themselves to being approached in this way. The mechanistic assumptions of the positivist and individualist traditions can pervade how all problems are formulated and approached by an organisation and coaching clients whose thinking is informed and shaped by these contexts.

An added, seductive, dimension here is that there are times when coachees and coaches may well get to feel as if they are at the top of their game in this regard. There are situations when it may well feel as if everything we are attempting is going to plan – where the world and all its complexity (at least at the surface of things and in the short term) is in alignment with our aspirations. This can feel wonderfully satisfying and reassuring as the anxiety associated with uncertainty and complexity is temporarily alleviated and we experience a congruence between the ego ideal and our action and impacts in the world.

Conversely, when faced with a situation that, given its complexity, defies instant understanding, or the identification of clear and effective action, coaches and coachees can experience anxiety, confusion, feelings of deficiency, loss of a sense of self esteem and agency, and sink into the corresponding and opposite state to omnipotence – that of impotence.

Impotence is a state of mind with corresponding beliefs and feelings of shame, inadequacy, helplessness, hopelessness, stuckness and absence of energy, potency or agency. The extent to which, through identification, we couple our sense of identity to our achievements, is the extent to which we also inevitably couple our sense of self to our limitations and inevitable failures in life. Instead of being able to befriend limitation and frame our experience as 'I am a person who has capacities and experience who simply was not able to make the best use of them this time', our only option is to see ourselves, aided and abetted by the superego's inner criticism, as a 'loser' or 'failure', with all the pain and contraction of potential that this entails.

Vulnerability – Befriending our humanity

One of the reasons why vulnerability and limitation are so difficult to bear is that we, as coaches and our coachees, are under enormous social pressure from the happiness imperative (Western, 2012) to be permanently positive and attain images and ideals of success and achievement. The pursuit of images becomes a series of imperatives or shoulds that keep us distanced from a deeper and more authentic sense of who we are and what we may genuinely desire, that is uniquely meaningful and purposeful to us.

Many writers on shame (Brown, 2013, 2015; Hollis, 2001; Kaufman, 1992) see vulnerability, however painful, as being very close to the authentic experience of being human.

Hollis (2001) points to the inevitability of human vulnerability and the way in which the goal of self-esteem based on the pursuit of images of success is yet another attempt to avoid the inevitable. This can give rise to an often unconscious expectation among coachees and coaches that development and learning should *always* move in the direction of quickly feeling better and more effective. There can be little room here for allowing and thinking about discomfort or the experience of limitation. Western (2012) describes how certain approaches to coaching can be oriented primarily towards fulfilling narcissistic ego ideals and advocates for an expansion in orientation through what he refers to as the 'soul guide discourse' to connect individuals to their deeper sense of self, vulnerabilities and true purpose.

For Brenne Brown (2013), being able to own and bear our vulnerability is key to experiencing ourselves, our emotions and our lives more fully and remaining creative in the face of challenges. While it is undoubtedly painful it is also 'the cradle of the emotions and experiences that we crave' (p. 34). If we defend against feeling vulnerable, we might avoid the dark, but we also deny ourselves the experience of the light. When it comes to closing down on our emotions we cannot be selective. Numbing the difficult inevitably results in a numbing of that which we desire. For Brown, 'vulnerability is the birthplace of love, belonging, joy, courage, empathy and creativity. It is the source of hope, empathy, accountability and authenticity' (p. 34).

Hollis (2001) points to the illusory nature of the pursuit of a self esteem which is based on living up to self-images and ego ideals – 'A person with high self-esteem is often one with a narcissistic personality disorder whose whole persona is devoted to hiding from others his or her secret emptiness' (p. 89). He goes on to say that

> anyone with a modicum of consciousness and a mild dollop of integrity will be able to enumerate a very long list of screw-ups, short-comings, betrayals, moments of cowardice and generalised incompetence. Anything less than a very long list suggests either an undeveloped awareness or an act of great self-deception.
>
> (p. 89)

Being realistic and open to acknowledging our limitations and shortcomings for Hollis 'seems to constitute the most modest level of conscious endeavour' (p. 89). This can also guard against the risk in organisational life of hubris – the fall from grandiosity eloquently described in the myth of Icarus.

Icarus's father Daedalus constructed wings to enable him and Icarus to escape from Crete. He warns his son to fly level – not too low, lest the dampness of the sea clog his wings (impotence), nor too high, lest the sun melt the wax holding the feathers together. The over ambitious Icarus, giddy on the thrill of flight and his ability (omnipotence), soars too close to the sun; his wings melt, and he plummets back to earth in catastrophic fashion.

Being grandiose extremes, ego ideals that are disconnected from a wider and more complex perspective on reality, both ends of the omnipotence/omniscience – impotence continuum are not as fixed or permanent as they can feel to be. It is never the case that we and our coachees know and can do everything. Nor is it ever the case, especially from an existential perspective, that there is nothing we know or nothing that we can do. Viktor Frankl brought this reality into stark relief in his book *Man's Search for Meaning* (2004). Here he describes how prisoners in the abominable conditions of German concentration camps in the Second World War all made choices about how to respond to conditions and treatment that they were powerless to change. What they were able to do was choose how they responded to this stark reality. He describes how some chose to give up, some made attempts at freedom which inevitably resulted in death, while others chose to find meaning in simple tasks, human relationship and the taking care of others. These pursuits seemed to provide meaning and sustenance and helped a number of people to survive.

From this, it would seem that, even where it appears that we are utterly helpless, we can always choose how to respond. Neurotic anxiety in the face of losing the illusion of control or an ego ideal can then give way to existential anxiety in the face of the unknown. This is the anxiety which we and our coachees need to learn to bear and contain if we are to stay open to making meaning, reflecting and creating new and timely responses to the different and complex challenges we and our clients face. In this way we develop the capacity to remain at the edge of chaos between the familiar and unknown long enough for new meaning and strategies to emerge.

Implicit in this process is mourning (Lapierre, 1993) the loss of omnipotent fantasies and ego ideals and an opening to the vulnerability and grace required to accept and live with that over which we have little or no control. The emphasis moves from trying to control the context to developing the flexibility to adjust and creatively choose our responses. It is in this response-ability that we take responsibility for creating the lives we live. As we and our coachees learn to understand shame, loosen identification with ideals and their impact on our experience and functioning, develop greater capacity individually and collectively to bear degrees of discomfort and exposure, it is more likely that we will be able to liberate ourselves from the tyranny of omnipotence and impotence and find ways to optimise our responses in the face of complexity, ambiguity and uncertainty.

In organisational life this can be particularly difficult given the pressures individuals find themselves under to have to aspire to omnipotence or omniscience in order to belong (and in the case of coaches in order to win work by promising predictable and extraordinary returns on investment). Coaches and coachees are vulnerable to the potent and primitive fear of rejection if they fail in some way. In the grip of these ideals, it can be hard to choose a path that feels simply 'good enough' and fit for a complex context. Anything short of the ideal is likely to be construed as mediocre rather than the best course of action in light of complex circumstances and what can and cannot be known at the time.

Example

A highly experienced learning and development professional, with a proven track record of delivering large scale culture change and leadership development projects, chose to question what he saw as the rather omnipotent fantasies of what his organisation's Board were seeking to achieve in a short timescale. He was told firmly by the CEO that 'thinking like that, you clearly don't have what it takes to work in this organisation'. The client came to coaching anxious about reputational damage and conflicted because his extensive experience to date suggested that what was being imagined was never going to be achieved in the timescale given a host of system dynamics and variables that also needed attention, and to which Board members appeared oblivious (or wilfully blind to in order to maintain their own ego ideals of omnipotence?). In his coaching he was able to come to understand the pressure in his organisation's culture for quick fixes and attachment to omnipotent fantasies. He was able to reign in his advocating a different perspective temporarily until Board members were able to arrive at their own conclusion, based on increasing evidence from the business, that things were not going to plan. This then enabled them to be more willing to listen to the coachee's perspectives and plot a more realistic and nonetheless successful course. In the process he also discovered he needed to reign in his own omnipotent fantasy that he could or should be able to quickly convince the Board of his perspectives, and was able to befriend his own limitations in that he could only facilitate their increased awareness of complexity at the pace that they could assimilate.

If we remove the maintenance of images and pursuit of specific ideals temporarily from the picture, the experience of omnipotence/omniscience (however disconnected from reality) enables us to feel our agency and capacity for creativity. The experience of impotence reminds us of there being limitation to our capacity, inevitable complexity and constraints in the external environment, and opens us to the experience of vulnerability. The difficulty is that when a coach or coachee is in the grip of ideals, these states become polarised and disconnected. In other words, omnipotence/omniscience is experienced as a state of capacity and knowledge that has no limits, whereas impotence is a state of total limitation without any possibility for creativity. Many clients and coaches will recognise the tendency to lurch between these two extremes. A session seemingly goes well and the coachee is delighted and we feel wonderful. Another session seemingly does not go well, the coachee does not arrive at any ground-breaking, profound insight, or impulse to take immediate and exceptional action, and we find ourselves going on an internal fault finding mission, telling ourselves we did a terrible job, imagining that any other coach would have been far more successful than us, and that this confirms us in a belief of fundamentally being not good enough. Comparison with others is often a signal that we are in the grip of our inner critic and shame experience. This movement is also a familiar one with coachees who have an extremely successful track record and then are promoted into a more complex role, where the strategies they have used in the past no longer work and where they may need to expand their perceptual frames and action logics in order to be successful. Their sense of self, based on past successes, is now threatened and they may experience self-doubt and confusion. There is a role here for coaching to normalise limitation, offer a container for anxiety and a reflective space for clients to learn and develop the capacity to adjust to the stretching requirements of their new context.

Furthermore, this lurching between omnipotence and impotence is mirrored in the 'heroes to zeros' culture that characterises many organisations, where coachees and coaches alike are fully aware that they are only seen to be as good as their last success, and where any perceived failure or limitation has the real potential to derail careers and dry up future engagements. Faced with this kind of pressure, coaches and coachees alike can become highly anxious about doing whatever is considered to be the right thing to fit in, even though this often is more ambiguous and unknown than appears to be the case. Doing what is seen to be wanted by the client and attempting to alleviate neurotic anxiety about getting it wrong takes the place of doing what might be required to contain existential anxiety in the face of not knowing how to proceed, and creating the possibility for creativity and discovery of different and more appropriate perspectives and behaviours.

At a three-day team meeting, the leader keeps telling the team coach 'we must be sure to end each day on a high!' – reflecting the anxiety clients can feel in the face of a more complex and wider range of human experience and the resulting pressure to manipulate feelings accordingly. At the end of the first day the team is in a subdued mood, having listened to a number of difficult messages about the health of the organisation and the financial and leadership challenges ahead. The leader takes the coach to one side and tells him that this is 'not the way' to end each day and they need to be more upbeat. The coach is able to say that he believes the team is understandably feeling deflated as they take in and digest the reality of their situation, and that any attempt at levity could be experienced as false and coercive. The coach trusts that by opening to the fuller and more complex realities of their situation, team members are likely to be more supported to find the resources they need in order to respond effectively than if they are made to feel that there is no room for emotion or vulnerability, and that they need to act at all times in accordance with an ideal of upbeat optimism. In spite of this, the coach has a rather anxious night in the face of the sponsor's anxiety and judgement that the coach is not providing the 'service' he wants. Fortunately, the second day begins with an open acknowledgement of the reality of the situation and team members begin to explore response strategies, becoming more energised and engaged as they recognise the need to collaborate in the face of the challenges they are facing together.

This example points to the possibility of there being a third position between omnipotence and impotence, where creativity and limitation can be held in creative tension rather than polarised. This is particularly suited to the complex challenges many clients face and can support clients to work through their identification with self-images and ego ideals. Where clients can be supported to see the way in which they lurch from one extreme position to the other and how this splits limitation and creativity, and therefore inflates each polarity to unrealistic proportions, they can begin to see that limitations, complexities and constraints in the environment do not have to imply (often unconsciously) limitation in themselves. If they can decouple their sense of themselves and worth from needing to be all powerful and successful in the environment, and learn to tolerate the vulnerability that comes from this, they can then also reconnect with a capacity for creativity in the face of more complex challenges.

The possibility arises that agency and worth are no longer connected to shoring up an image or idea, as when the client in the example above puts pressure on the coach to end on a high, in order presumably to support an idea of good leadership being equated with the team feeling upbeat and motivated. Instead, agency becomes associated with the experience, potential pleasure and satisfaction of working something through, as when the team members, through acknowledging their authentic experience of flatness in the face of situational challenges, and supported to contain anxiety by their coach, were able to come together and strategise effectively. As Hollis (2001) puts it 'if one is busy pursuing what needs to be pursued, is interested in something worthy, and finding it all getting more and more interesting, then one has scant time to brood on the pseudo-issue of self esteem' (p. 89).

This stands in marked contrast to teams where individual anxiety in the face of failure to live up to ideals of potency and capacity leads team members to compete internally with one another rather than collaborate or make relevant meaning together leading to more timely, coordinated and effective action.

This capacity to remain creative, interested and connected to the range of one's resources in the face of internal and external limitations is a key quality for responding to the challenges many clients face. Lapierre (1993) refers to this as a position of 'relative potency', where we feel we can still function and bring our reflexivity and creativity to bear in complex situations. Often this involves a process of mourning the loss of an illusory identity (through identification) that has been bound up with particular grandiose fantasies, self-images or ego ideals. As mindful awareness increases in both coachees and coaches about how they identify with particular images and how this feels, then identification tends to relax and we and our coachees can come to locate our sense of self more in the different capacities (including capacity to reflect) we can draw on in different situations to make sense of and navigate complexity and limitation, rather than in images that have to be maintained at all costs.

It also requires that we be able to bear vulnerability and normalise it. It is inevitable that when we experience failure in living up to an ideal we are likely to feel vulnerable and ashamed. Rather than defend against this through cynicism or disengagement, we need to be able to bear our vulnerability and go on thinking and acting. If we cannot decouple our sense of self from our self images and corresponding successes and achievements, then there is too much at stake for us to share our raw talents and gifts. We will not be able to risk getting it wrong for fear of experiencing shame which in turn erodes our tolerance for vulnerability and suffocates the possibility of human connection, trust, engagement, innovation, creativity and productivity – the very qualities complex situations call for in order to discover new and creative responses. Laloux (2014) sees 'taming the fears of the ego' (p. 44) as a quality that characterises a more expanded individual and collective corporate consciousness. He puts it thus, by

> looking at our ego from a distance, we can suddenly see how its fears, ambitions, and desires often run our life. We can learn to minimize our need for control, to look good, to fit in. We are no longer fused with our ego, and we don't let its fears reflexively control our lives

(p. 44)

He goes on to say that when we are fused with our egos, we are motivated and driven to make decisions on the basis of external factors such as what will others think or what specific outcomes can be achieved? As we learn to disidentify from the ego we start to orient more to our emerging sense of our own inner guidance and internal compass. We now become concerned with the question of 'inner rightness: does this decision seem right? Am I being true to myself? Is this in line with who I sense I'm called to become? Am I being of service to the world?' (p. 44). With fewer ego-based fears we can develop the capacity to experiment and take decisions that may feel riskier or where we have not, or are simply unable to, weigh up all the possible outcomes but, nonetheless, need to take action. In this way

> we develop a sensitivity for situations that don't feel quite right, situations that demand that we speak up and take action, even in the face of opposition or with seemingly low odds of success, out of a sense of integrity and authenticity. Recognition, success, wealth, and belonging are viewed as pleasureable experiences, but also as tempting traps for the ego . . . we do not pursue recognition, success, wealth, and belonging to live a good life. We pursue a life well-lived, and the consequences might just be recognition, success, wealth and love.
>
> (pp. 44–45)

Practice considerations

As we have set out in this chapter, failure (real or imagined) to live up to personal and organisational ideals of omnipotence and omniscience can give rise to the experience of shame, as can failure to comply with those cultural and behavioural expectations in a particular organisational context that confer belonging and membership. The inhibiting effects of shame do not only operate in relation to policing extremes of behaviour, which would obviously be damaging to a human system, but also act as a force for maintaining the status quo and adherence to organisation norms which might legitimately need questioning and relaxing in order for necessary experimentation and effective change to occur.

In this book we have been proposing that a relational orientation to coaching offers the possibility to explore the relationship the client has to her organisation. From a complexity perspective, in order for individual and organisational change and development to occur, the forces for control and homogeneity have to be held in dynamic tension with space to imagine and explore difference and alternative possibilities, some of which may challenge current orthodoxies and received wisdom. Whenever a coachee is faced with considering something that moves away from alignment with the 'parent' organisation's existing norms, it is possible that shame and anxiety related to membership, belonging and reputation will be evoked.

As a result of its deeply private and painful nature, recognising and working with shame can be a delicate and subtle process. A tension needs to be held between having an understanding of shame phenomena and working to reduce these, and the very real shaming potential of overtly or prematurely drawing attention to them with our coachees who might then feel overly exposed.

A relational orientation to practice, with sensitive attunement to the co-creation of experience between coach and coachee, is well suited to working with shame phenomena. As the experience of shame is so intricately bound up with the need for human connection and being accepted, along with anxiety related to being unwelcome or considered to be deficient and lacking in some way, the most fundamental antidote to shame is the quality of the relationship between coach and coachee.

Offering a supportive, authentic and attuned orientation to clients; tracking the levels of support a client has to sit with uncertainty; normalising vulnerability, anxiety and self-doubt; educating clients about the shame based nature of our 'inner critic'; being willing to talk of our own experience of limitation; offering an attitude of compassion and acceptance with space and permission for clients to bring more of their experience than just that which supports images of success and competence, all stand to create conditions in which coachees might come to feel less burdened by their anxiety.

Brenne Brown (2013) stresses the inevitability of emotional exposure and vulnerability, attempting to avoid them is pointless. For her, the only option we have is for engagement with our vulnerability as this will determine the depth of our courage. If as coaches we cannot open to these experiences in ourselves, we are not likely to authentically be able to meet others in theirs. Furthermore, the relationship can offer opportunities for anxiety to be explored and contained in order for new thinking to emerge. This can be demanding for coaches who need to have learnt to bear their own existential anxiety in the face of not knowing what might happen next or what use the client might be able to put them to. If a coach is concerned with image, she is more likely to be preoccupied with having a specific impact rather than discovering with each client how she might be of service. In the words of Brenne Brown, working with shame processes requires coaches to 'dare greatly' in facing their own vulnerability and also take a stand against the dominance of the individualist paradigm, managerial and organisational discourses which deny emotion and vulnerability.

Again this can be particularly challenging because coachees in the grip of anxiety can look to coaches to rescue. Adam Phillips (1997) explores how, wherever there is anxiety and uncertainty that feels too much to bear, we tend to look for 'experts' to alleviate our suffering. This means that coaches can be under powerful projective pressure also to 'do' something. Particularly if we have not developed the capacity to bear our own anxiety and contain the fear of being rejected if we are not instantly and consistently made use of by the client. We can resort to tools, models and grandiose promises to attempt to alleviate anxiety, finding ourselves getting busy and having an increasing investment in getting the client somewhere, or proving to them that we are useful (yet another manifestation of the individualist paradigm). We might even find ourselves wanting to move quickly to educate our clients about anxiety and shame to try to get them 'over' it.

Instead, working with a sensitivity to shame calls for adopting a more gentle and indirect orientation where as coaches we might hint at shame processes in language that a client might be able to relate to. With a client who is talking of feeling anxious about his appraisal because of not having delivered on a project due to a host of extraneous difficulties, we might find a way of saying something like:

'I can really understand how in your competitive culture you might be feeling a little anxious right now. It seems to me that there is not a lot of room in your organisation to reflect on the wider causes of difficulties other than holding individuals to account or blaming them when things don't go to plan.'

This intervention serves to communicate attunement to the coachee by the coach, conferring an experience of being understood in a non-judgemental way. It also points to the wider context in which the coachee works and the influence of context in shaping individual experience.

By widening in this way the perspective on the coachee's situation he may feel supported not to take all the responsibility upon himself and come to view his situation and experience in a more contextualised way. From an individualistic perspective this strategy might be viewed as a 'cop out' in relation to responsibility, but it is our experience that when more of the total situation and factors contributing to a coachees's experience are taken into consideration, people are more likely to be able to take *greater* responsibility for the part they have played and do something about it. It is far easier to take a manageable and accurate portion of responsibility when we are not feeling burdened with all the blame (whether this is done to us or we do it to ourselves). Some coachees may have a tendency to take on all the responsibility even when this is not the case and this tendency can also be explored in the coaching relationship.

A relational orientation to coaching, where coaches make themselves more present and available to be impacted by clients, empathise, share their own vulnerability at times, and how they have been touched by another human being, can act as a powerful connective antidote to shame experience which is profoundly bound up with actual or imagined disconnection. The implicit relational domain which we described in Section 2 is key here. Being able to sit with not knowing with an other, and experience a coach being calm and thoughtful in the face of uncertainty, can regulate anxiety in the coachee and models a way of remaining resourced in the face of not knowing that does not involve rushing to action.

Over time coachees can internalise the experience of the coach and the support and reflexivity they experience, laying down new neural networks that they can activate for themselves in challenging situations outside of the coaching room. This stands to shift the source of identity and self experience from being located in the realm of internal images to the experiential territory of participation, curiosity, discovery and meaning making.

In summary

Working to reduce shame, develop shame resilience and tame the ego through disidentification with ego ideals is key to:

- Enabling greater acceptance of self, other and contextual complexities.
- Relaxing the investment in taking up and defending positions in order to be 'right', which inevitably requires that any other perspective must be made 'wrong'.
- Opening more to inquiry, understanding and dialogue.
- Facilitating greater collaborative meaning making and action informed by deeper understanding of more of the total situation and context.
- Supporting greater respectful questioning of the status quo.
- Enabling greater risk and daring in thinking beyond current or received wisdom, leading to the generation of more options for action.
- Greater support for innovation, informed experimentation, agility and responsiveness.

Chapter 10

Perspectives on contracting from a relational perspective

Contracting for and framing coaching engagements are generally agreed to be fundamental processes in ensuring productive and effective coaching interventions. This is further supported by research into coaching effectiveness which points to the importance of sufficient shared agreement between relevant parties in relation to objectives for the work (Clutterbuck and David, 2013). From within an individualistic and rationalist paradigm, there seems to be an assumption in some literature that this is a relatively straightforward process where it is assumed that all parties are clear, rational and cooperative in this exercise.

A relational orientation, and practice experience, would suggest that this is not necessarily the case. More intersubjective and relational views of an organisation as a complex adaptive system of human interaction (Cavanagh, 2006; Stacey, 2001), where meaning and the organisation itself are being constructed, maintained or changed via the medium of conversations, suggest that beneath the surface of apparently reasoned and collaborative conversations there can be many dynamics at play which can impact and affect the tone, climate, boundaries, direction and outcome of coaching. Field (Parlett, 1991) and complexity perspectives (Eoyang and Holladay, 2013) also point to the interconnectedness and mutually influencing properties of multiple factors in determining how individuals experience themselves and behaviours arise.

Contracting – Who are the parties?

A relational perspective is oriented to an appreciation of intersubjectivity and the implicit differences in the ways in which individuals construct reality. As such, contracting from this perspective involves working out together how a particular intervention may be being co-constructed by all involved parties, accepting and acknowledging that, while there may be areas of shared understanding and intention, there will just as likely be areas of difference which may need to be surfaced, acknowledged and negotiated. An added level of complexity is that these differences are not always articulated or visible in the public conversations which take place at the initial contracting stage or in the organisation in general. Often they are hidden from the public arena, but make themselves felt in the coaching relationship and in interactions the coach might have with stakeholders during the course of the work. Coachees also often use the coaching relationship to make public with the coach beliefs, aspirations and perspectives that they would not wish others in the organisation to know, and yet which inevitably have an impact on their taking up of their role. Charlotte Sills (2012) talks of the coaching contract as fundamentally acknowledging that there is a 'me' and a 'you', representing two subjectivities in relationship. She goes on to say that in making contracts 'we are facing the existential reality that we are separate and different and we may have different desires – and yet we are also connected and can join in mutual commitment' (p. 94). She says that, at best, coaching engages with the challenge of this existential encounter of how to join in the full acceptance and knowledge of differences. This tension operates at the individual level and between coach, coachee and stakeholders, and mirrors the tension at the organisational level between sameness and difference, structure and emergence, order and chaos.

Human beings have a need to impose structure and order to a complex and changing world. This helps to reduce anxiety. At the same time, the pseudo-security derived in this way can limit growth and learning in the face of complex and novel challenges, as we tend to apply what we already know to a situation that might actually be calling for the development of new learning and different strategies to those we have become used to. Stacey (1992) refers to the space between order and chaos as the area of 'bounded instability', which Sills (2012) describes as 'a sort of temporary beneficial disorder that allows for something new to emerge' (p. 95). How individual coaches and clients negotiate and hold these tensions will depend on many variables including the background and preferences of the coach and personality characteristics of all, as well as the multitude of forces at work in the organisation at that particular time which may put pressure on coaches and coachees alike to lean more towards one end of the order-chaos continuum. The individualist, rationalist and positivist biases of many organisations lead individuals to see the world primarily in terms of predictability and control. Relationally oriented coaches who believe in the value of bounded instability in service of transformational learning have to tread a fine line between meeting the organisation where it is in relation to control, while simultaneously providing sufficient novelty and difference to catalyse learning and change. Furthermore, coachees developing new insights and capacities in the context of coaching will need to negotiate and work out how to deploy new perspectives and intentions within the dominant ideologies, culture and ways of working that are established in the organisation.

Contours of contracting

Sills (2012) gives a detailed overview of the different levels at which contracting can operate and these are summarised in the table below:

Level/Type of Contract	Focus
Level 1	
With the wider world, society planet	Establishing those basic principles and values that will not be transgressed i.e. no harm to others or the planet.
Level 2	
With the organisation and its parts	Transparent clarification of expectations between coachee, coach and organisational representatives i.e. line managers, HR Department.
Administrative contract	Clarify practical arrangements such as number, duration, location and frequency of sessions; fee and cancellation policy; confidentiality and its limits.
Professional learning or development contract	Define purpose and focus of coaching 'what, so what, now what?'
Level 3	
Contracting with coaching client/coachee	Establish the goals of the work and the tasks involved. Establish the direction of the work 'what?' and how coach and coachee will be with one another. Explore how the coachee frames and understands the presenting issues. Contract for the coaching relationship and how to manage difficulties that might arise. Identify whether goals are hard or soft. (See below.)
Level 4	
Sessional contract	Establishing the focus and process of each session.
Level 5	
Moment by moment contract	Negotiating moment by moment with the coachee on how to proceed; establishing permission to share an observation, information or design an experiment; negotiating and seeking permission to explore the impact of a micro exchange between coach and coachee 'what happened just then?'; negotiating to move out of content and review the process of the session.

Types of contract

Sills (2012) goes on to identify four types of contract with the coachee based on two intersecting variables. One continuum is that between a 'hard' contract where the intended goals are observable and verifiable as in 'to introduce a new performance management process to my team' and the 'soft' contract which allows the unknown to emerge, is more subjective and less specific as in 'to understand my leadership style better'. The other continuum is based on whether the client and coach know where the client currently is and the changes he or she wishes to make. This gives rise to the following four possible types of contract:

Clarifying – where the frame is a hard contract, specific and verifiable, but where the client does not yet know precisely the changes he or she wishes or needs to make.

Exploratory – where the frame is soft, subjective and where the client does not know the changes he or she wishes or needs to make.

Growth and discovery – where the frame is soft and where the client does have a sense of the changes he or she wishes to make.

Behavioural outcome – where the frame is a hard focus and the client knows the changes he or she wishes or needs to make.

Goals – Defining and constraining.

From a relational perspective where meaning emerges in the context of a conversation over time, goals can raise a number of challenges. Goals can bring clarity and focus, helping to orient the coach and coachee to the individual needs and hopes of the coachee and context requirements. At the same time, they can constrain imagination, possibility and exploration if they are held too tightly (Grant, 2013). Here they can result in the field of possibility becoming narrow, where data and phenomena are selected by both coach and a coachee for attention or discounted on the basis of often unspoken assumptions about the relevance of coachee material to the attainment of stated goals. Goals can only ever be an aspiration imagined and experienced in the present moment. It is never possible to know if that which we imagine, when we get it, is actually what we might want, like or what might be needed in context. Goals can also be shaped in or out of conscious awareness by the forces and pressures of the context and other stakeholders, so the coachee's own relationship to goals is never really explored. It is all too often assumed that goals can be taken at face value. Holding goals lightly, and monitoring them regularly for progress and continued relevance, will serve to keep the space for possibilities and discovery open.

Relational, intersubjective and contextual dynamics of contracting

Whatever contract is agreed upon with the coachee, contracting in organisations takes place in a context where there will be a range of different stakeholders involved explicitly and implicitly with the contracting process and outcomes of the coaching. This can influence the coachee and subtly, and not so subtly, affect the field conditions in which the coaching is taking place. Given the indivisibility, from a relational perspective, of individual and context, these field conditions cannot but contribute to an individual's learning and behavioural outcomes.

Skinner (2012) describes how the relationship coaches have with their coachees is inevitably influenced by relationship dynamics outside of the coaching dyad that find their way with varying degrees of conscious awareness and force into the coaching relationship.

A relational orientation to coaching is inclined towards attending to these forces wherever possible, as they can have a significant impact on the quality of relating, learning and growth. Furthermore, relationships with other stakeholders as perceived, imagined, constructed in the mind of both coach and coachee can subtly and profoundly influence the co-created dynamics of the coaching relationship as well as, at times, being the very focus of the coaching conversations themselves. Skinner (2012) points out that business realities mean that a coach may find himself sharing relationships with the same multi-party stakeholders within the organisation as the coachee they are working with. In addition, coaches might also bring, with varying degrees of awareness, into the coaching room their own aspirations, fears and fantasies related to these stakeholders. It can be immensely challenging for coaches not to be concerned about 'getting results' for a demanding and highly influential stakeholder. If these contextual preoccupations infiltrate the coach-coachee relationship too strongly, then it can have a marked influence on the coach's ability to be in service of the coachee and hold a more spacious and open stance to the work, in order for the coachee to discover their own learning, meanings and strategies for action. We frequently supervise coaches whose capacity for allowing the coaching process to unfold has at times been constrained by an often unconscious desire to please the stakeholder (often in order to secure more work) over and above being in service of the coachee and their context.

Coaches have to hold a tension of being in the service of both the coachee and the organisation sponsoring and paying for the work. Skinner (2012) sets out a number of dynamics related to organisational politics that can have a bearing upon the coaching relationship. These include:

Multiple accountabilities

This is where line executives supporting the coaching of their chosen coachees have an investment in outcome for the coachee and the performance of their own department or function, as well as the executive meeting requirements of his or her people development role. Thus coach and coachee are also working in service of the executive fulfilling aspects of his or her own contract with the organisation.

Different understanding about goals, coaching methods, processes and outcomes

Line managers and sponsors of coaching may not be as knowledgeable about the methodologies, scope and practices of coaching as the coach. This can lead to a host of differences in relation to expectations of what might be desirable, realistic and the timescale required for change to occur. Furthermore, stakeholders' assumptions about change, often steeped in linear and mechanistic principles, may incline them to a narrower goal and specific behaviour outcome focus which may not necessarily be relevant to the coachee or optimal given the context.

Preoccupation with impact

Others in the organisation might perceive that they might be impacted either positively or negatively by any behavioural changes or changes the coachee chooses to make in how he relates to the organisation. Depending on what they imagine to be at stake, their personalities, levels of awareness and seniority, they might either act in ways that undermine the coachee fulfilling their potential or in ways that stand for and facilitate the coachee's success.

Shifting sands

The volatility and turbulence of much organisational life and economic/market forces might lead to rapidly changing perceptions of the coachee's business performance, even though many of the factors contributing to a reduction in performance may be out of the individual's control.

Time and logistics related subtexts

Time pressures can lead line executives to sponsor or initiate coaching activities for reasons that may not be overtly and transparently named, but which nonetheless can subtly and powerfully influence the coach-coachee-stakeholder relationship. Where these sub-texts might actually be more compelling to sponsors and executives than the overt contract, coach and coachee might find their work and relationship characterised by confusion and mixed messages.

Executives commissioning the services of a coach often bring the taken for granted assumption that coaching will quickly persuade their direct report to behave in a way that better meets or exceeds their performance expectations (Skinner, 2012). Furthermore, there can be an assumption that the executive knows what is needed and knows what is best for the organisation. This orientation stems from the positivist and individualist tradition that many organisations still operate within. This can deny or limit the potential for coach and coachee to discover new ways in which performance might be increased that might actually differ from the expectations of the person commissioning the work. These might actually be more effective and motivating for the coachee and may unlock potential and interrupt negative patterns in the wider organisation. These differences in perception will need to be aired, explored and negotiated in and outside of the coaching dyad.

An added dimension is the personality types and interpersonal styles of all stakeholders including HR and Learning and Development Managers which can have a bearing on how the practicalities and objectives of coaching are negotiated and positioned (Sills and Wide, 2006 cited in Skinner, 2010). Different preferences such as for affiliation or personal recognition on the part of the line manager can make for very different system dynamics. In the former case, the line manager is more likely to work collaboratively with HR and Learning and Development functions and be interested in understanding and ensuring that agreed processes are adhered to. In the latter case, a line manager might be inclined to operate more as a maverick, using their positional authority to push through the commissioning of a coach with scant regard for organisational processes and procedures (Skinner,

2012). In the former case, it is likely that consultation might make for more alignment and goodwill in the system, which in turn finds its way into supporting the coaching intervention. In the latter, the field conditions are likely to be characterised by greater difference and even competitive hostility which, again, is likely to make itself felt to both coach and coachee and call for sensitive negotiation.

Enter the coach

From the examples above it can be seen that once we open to considering the intersubjective and relational dimensions of an organisation (the CONTEXT of the coach-coachee-context constellation) in how we think about coaching and contracting, the field becomes more complex but also, potentially, more creative. Complexity and diversity bring greater opportunities for enabling stakeholders and coachees to be open to multiple perspectives and intelligences, thereby generating potentially more timely and effective strategies that factor in more of the dynamics of the total situation in which the coaching is occurring. Coaches working from a relational and systemic orientation need to be as attentive to the dynamics of the coach-coachee-context constellation as they are to the specifics of the coach-coachee dyad.

In this context, credibility, authority and future work for the coach come not from accreditation credentials alone, but from how a coach actually engages with and finds ways with the coachee to effectively navigate this complexity. Skinner (2012) proposes that if coaches use information about the organisation in mutually beneficial ways, they are more likely to be trusted by clients and stakeholders. He highlights that one way to collapse and manage the intersubjective tensions outlined above is to adhere to rigid rules, protocols and positions as a coach. In practice, however, coaching requires coaches increasingly to navigate greater and greater complexity. This mirrors the ways in which coachees in organisations are often having to manage greater and greater complexity, where fixed ideas and 'yesterday's learning' is no longer fit for purpose. Coachees increasingly have to read the situation they find themselves in, in the full know-ledge that they will never be able to see or understand all the factors influencing the field, reflect, generate options and take a risk to commit to action, the out-comes of which can never be fully predicted and may create unintended ripples throughout the organisation – ripples which can both be problematic and generative.

Skinner (2012) describes how, despite their best intentions

> any coach would be naïve to believe they can simply establish some kind of three-way contract . . . once and for all at the beginning of a relationship with an executive in a large organisation – and then be left alone to manage it without external interference.

> (p. 118)

Intervening in the system – Contracting as a complex adaptive conversation

The more coaches develop a relational orientation that factors in the dynamics and complexities of context, the more they may find themselves intervening in the stakeholder system in which the coaching is taking place. Contracting and subsequent conversations between coach, coachee and stakeholders offer a context in which a number of the challenges and tensions named so far might be surfaced and the context impacted in order to create conditions in which coaching might be successful and supported (although specific success measures might not always be able to be defined in advance).

From an integrative and relational perspective, coaches and their clients are involved in the negotiation, construction, monitoring and reworking of a working alliance (contract) that will be impacted by and reflect the complexity, variables and dynamics at play in the context/situation that the coach is working in, as well as the personality, training and background of the coach. In this sense contracting can be seen as a process of collaborative meaning making between coach, coachee and stakeholders (context). It is likely always to be partial, in that not all that is occuring in a human system, or the meanings that operate within it, can ever be seen or understood at once. When relationship dynamics and differences emerge in ways that impact the coaching, all participants in the coaching intervention have an opportunity to consider and explore these differences for what they might have to offer in terms of learning both within and beyond the boundaries of the coaching dyad.

This is a challenge to linear and positivist assumptions about organisations. It is not possible to see all the dynamics influencing conversations and behaviour in an organisation nor try to control them, furthermore they are likely to be fluid and shifting. Coaches need to hold meanings and perspectives lightly and respond reflectively in real time to events as they arise. This mirrors the situational reflection- in-action orientation of a relational approach to coaching and is a fractal reflecting how change happens from a complexity perspective. In this way the coach stands to model what coachees might also need to develop in themselves for navigating the complexities of their contexts.

Developing a relational orientation and the trust required for managing contracting complexities happens and is refined over time. The multitude of variables in any coach-coachee-context constellation will throw up particular challenges, and different ways to hold and navigate tensions will be different each time. This is at once the challenge *and* the source of creativity, excitement and satisfaction of working in this way, and why supervision is essential support for practicing with this orientation.

Skinner (2012) sets out a number of pragmatic ways to navigate the complexity of various multi-party stakeholders and differing expectations. His intention is that this should be in service of maximising the value and ethical maturity of coaching practice and the profession. These include coaches:

- Fully recognising that they have a professional duty both to the organisational client providing the funding as well as to the individual coachee. This may be a source of tension that needs to be held, explored and worked with.
- Approaching multi-party contracting as a continuing and evolving process requiring vigilance and regular re-negotiation with interested parties to maintain alignment in ever shifting contexts.
- Developing their self-awareness so they can recognise and better manage their own perceptual, emotional and behavioural patterns. From a relational perspective these resonances in the coach are likely to contain rich information about particular forces in the context and how the coach is being impacted by them. Coaches need to pay close attention to how they respond to the stresses and temptations they might experience when dealing with complex, politically charged dilemmas.
- Working to identify key external stakeholders and understand as much as possible about their business as well as personal interests, perspectives, personality and patterns that might have a bearing on the framing, execution and outcome of the coaching engagement.
- Taking account of the personal style and behavioural preferences of stakeholders where possible. This may be through direct observation, but also on the basis of how they are referred to by the coachee and 'imagined' in the coaching dyad. This can support tentative meaning making about the probable intent as well as the impact of those stakeholders on the coaching relationship.
- Recognising and surfacing for discussion, at an early stage, any implicit expectation by external stakeholders that the coaching will be used to persuade or coerce the coachee. Skinner (2012) stresses that the coach should not take personal responsibility to 'protect' the coachee from this attempted persuasion – coachees might well choose to be persuaded to perform in a certain way if they feel this is in line with legitimate corporate expectations and might support their career aspirations and progression. The coach's role is to explore the implications of this both in relation to the coachee and stakeholder expectations and what might be possible.
- Maintaining focus primarily on adding value through support for learning and growth in the coachee and client organisation, avoiding over-attachment to their own process preferences or future business-development opportunities.
- Monitoring and raising for discussion first with the coachee any perception of external interference that either party considers as having a negative impact on the progress of the coaching relationship.

> • Using supervision to be attentive for any boundary blurring or violations they may feel coerced or tempted into committing through the application of external influence and be willing to consider these pulls as data from the field.
>
> (Adapted from Skinner, 2012)

Skinner (2012) goes on to encourage coaches to consider that their work involves making an intervention into a complex adaptive system where a multitude of forces will be applied continuously from outside the coaching room on both the coach and coachee. He proposes that a coach does not serve stakeholders well by simply adhering with positive intent to rigid boundaries or codes of conduct and not engaging with relationships outside of the coaching room. This is because business realities and human systems dynamics frequently cause stakeholders to behave in unexpected ways, not necessarily the way the coach feels, or codes of conduct imply they 'should'.

Paying attention to boundary dynamics

As we have set out earlier, relational perspectives view the self and self experience as having dynamic properties which shift according to the field conditions at any time and the ways in which these are engaged with by individuals. From this perspective it could be argued that coach and coachee are in a process of meaning making and self-construction influenced by their individual preferences, backgrounds and the organisation context in which the coaching is taking place. One implication of this perspective is that coaches need also to consider the nature of boundary phenomena between coach, coachee and context. We revisit some of the perspectives set out in Chapter 4 with specific relevance for contracting.

Individual – Organisation

Coaching, by the process of being a one to one intervention in a context, raises the tension of the individual and organisation. As we have described above, the coachee's agenda for development and personal interest may align or diverge in varying degrees from the organisation's agenda as embodied by stakeholders, leaders and those commissioning coaching services. A number of individual-to-context relationship dynamics are possible here.

Coachee to context

Different recipients of coaching will be differently disposed toward the intervention We have discussed earlier how attachment theorists have identified that early patterns of interaction with caregivers establish very strong and unconscious patterns of expectation and interaction in human relationships, which also translate over into work relationships and the relationship to the organisation itself. As a result of these psychological patternings, some coachees will be inclined to comply unquestioningly with the requirements of the context, while others may appear to have an almost allergic reaction to any expectation of stakeholders, experiencing them as unacceptable demands, and reacting with passive-aggressive resistance or outright hostility.

The same possibilities (along with a myriad of graded positions between the two extremes) also apply to coaches and organisational stakeholders. Acknowledging and exploring these dynamics can create possibilities for adjustments that are in the interests of all parties. Without this perspective there is a risk of position-taking on all sides and differences being construed as needing to be neutralised or rebelled against.

Coach to context

Some coaches will be more inclined, with varying degrees of conscious awareness, to view the organisation as an authority to be obeyed. Others may be more inclined to surface and explore questions of power and authority and how these might be informing the way in which the coaching contract is being co-constructed in the minds of all participants involved in commissioning the work, including the coachee.

Career background and orientation also play an important part here. Coaches who have come to coaching after long corporate careers may be more identified with organisation culture and the need for compliance in service of predictability, belonging and control. Career coaches and organisation consultants who have been tasked for many years to ask provocative questions in service of organisational development and transformational learning may find it easier to question. Professional survival, reputational anxiety and financial concern also contribute to informing the position a coach might take on the individual-organisation continuum.

Stakeholder to context

Different stakeholders (the line manager, department head etc.) may also come with different values and perspectives on learning and development. Some will be very motivated by concern for homogeneity, control and containment, where others might be more comfortable with an ontological orientation, surfacing and questioning the basic assumptions that govern the construction of the organisation's reality and behaviour, and that may also be implicated in the challenges the organisation currently faces.

Public – Private

Psychoanalytic (Gould *et al.*, 2001; Hirschhorn, 1993) perspectives on organisational life point to the complex human system dynamics which operate 'under the surface' in organisations and shape patterns of human interaction. When contracting with coachees and organisation stakeholders, what is said publicly may not be precisely what is meant or desired. Yet more linear and mechanistic assumptions about organisations being predominantly rational and logical would take this at face value. Coaches and coachees often have to manage the differences that exist in the public narratives that are being constructed and the more private realities that often reveal themselves in the confidential context of the coaching relationship.

Control – Emergence

More managerial and 'rational' approaches to OD and coaching are predicated on assumptions of cause and effect and the logical sequencing between interventions and predictable outcomes (Cavicchia, 2009). This can give rise to coaching where the coach works to maintain focus tightly within the parameters set by the organisation. This may be appropriate and useful where skills development is the focus of the work and all parties are in sufficient agreement and alignment as to the scope and objectives of the intervention. The measure of success can be predicted, sought and may even be quantified.

Such an approach becomes more problematic where the coachee may be needing to use coaching as a reflective space to explore and make sense of the challenges she faces, the impacts of these on her identity, self image and efficacy, in order to develop the resources and resilience to respond to complex situations in creative and effective ways. Here it is more difficult to predict precisely what use the coachee will be able to make of the coaching intervention, as transformational learning involving a shift in internal perceptual frames, is by its very nature, relatively unpredictable and difficult to identify or know from within an existing frame of reference.

As a result of this, coaches may wish to raise questions or explore these dynamics at the early stages of stakeholder conversations. Questions like:

- What might the implications be if the coachee cannot or does not want to make the changes deemed necessary?
- How is information about the system to be fed back and thought about between all parties?
- What forces at work in the context or system might have a bearing on the agency and potential success of the coachee?
- What might need to change in how stakeholders interact with the coachee and his or her context in order to support his or her efficacy and success?

These questions can provide a number of possibilities, they can:

- Reveal information about organisation and interpersonal dynamics that might have a bearing on the coaching engagement.
- Allow paradoxes and tensions to be surfaced and explored.
- Initiate new and different conversations in the stakeholder group and wider organisation.
- Sensitise the organisation to the relationship between individual behaviour, performance and system dynamics.
- Potentially influence the field conditions to be more supportive of the coachee's development, or at least alert all parties to what may or may not be realistic to expect.
- Allow stakeholders to have a direct experience of how the coach embodies and makes use of a relational and contextual orientation to practice.

Example

The following brief example is just one way in which such tensions can arise and be responded to by coach and coachee.

A recently promoted leader in a very male dominated organisation had been told in an appraisal that she needed to 'toughen up and be more authoritative'. Every time she spoke of this her voice became almost inaudible and she would break eye contact and look down. The coach sensed that the client might be feeling vulnerable and exposed in relation to the issue of her authority and feeling some pain at the directness of the feedback she had received. The coachee went on talking about feeling she needed to make progress fast and 'just get on with it', but it was clear to the coach that her heart was not in the work. At this point the coach remembered that earlier the client had said with some distaste that she experienced many leaders in the organisation as 'bullying'. Furthermore, organisational performance was deteriorating and employee satisfaction surveys had revealed for a number of years an alarming downward trend in employee motivation attributed to a climate of intimidation. In a gentle, clear and simultaneously matter of fact tone the coach speculated aloud . . .

'I can appreciate the pressure you might be feeling to get a quick result given the pace of your organisation and the operational challenges you face. It's tricky isn't it? You have been told you need to be authoritative and feel this doesn't come easily to you, added to which, you might not want to use authority in the way you see others using it. I wonder if our challenge might be to explore what type of authority you might be able and willing to develop in yourself and use with your team . . . how does that sound to you?'

At this point the coachee looked up and was able to hold eye contact as she said, 'Yeah, that's it, I know I need to be more assertive, but I really don't want to be like my boss!' This began a fruitful conversation that ended ultimately in the coachee embodying a way of being authoritative that met the requirements of her role without compromising her own values and personality style. Over time this resulted in performance improvements in the coachee's team that also attracted positive attention from colleagues and senior leaders. The organisation is now involved in addressing the highly pressured culture and attempting to introduce greater equilibrium between operational imperatives and employee inclusion and engagement.

Chapter 11

Coaching in organisations

Culture, norms and novelty

How we think about organisations, and the assumptions we hold about how they work, inevitably affects how we view coaching clients, their contexts, how change might be facilitated and what challenges there may be for clients and coaches alike. The positivist and individualist traditions give rise to a series of working assumptions that persist in many organisations to this day.

These assumptions and the patterns of thinking and acting that flow from them are maintained by organisation members who shape them and are shaped by them. System and relational perspectives demonstrate how patterns of practice and norms shape the social construction of individual realities. Change often involves individuals daring to think differently to established norms and the courage to publicly experiment with new knowledge and strategies, a process Western (2017, 2012) refers to as disrupting the normative.

In this chapter we shall describe a number of normative forces which can be seen to be at work in organisations. They represent working assumptions, biases and orientations which powerfully shape how individuals perceive the world, feel and think. We have used the metaphor of 'forces' to emphasise the inevitable relationship between perception, feeling and thinking and the possibilities for action they either enable or constrain.

Objectivity and the rational

Many organisation theorists have now commented on the tendency in organisations to privilege the rational (De Vries, 2001; Czander, 1993; Hirschhorn & Barnett, 1993; Morgan, 1986; Obholzer & Zagier-Roberts, 1994; Stacey, 2001; Western, 2017, 1012). This is, in part, due to the early establishment of scientific paradigms (Gilbreth, 1911; Taylor, 1911), predicated on mind-body dualism (Wheeler, 2000) as dominant lenses for studying and intervening in organisations, coupled with the anxiety that can be evoked when considering the complexity of human subjectivity, intersubjectivity and the unpredictability this gives rise to.

In its extreme forms, organisational rationality attempts to completely deny any subjective and emotional life, turning organisations into what Morgan (1986) has termed 'psychic prisons'. Tasks and processes are privileged over dialogue and reflection, the cognitive over the affective, doing over being.

The bias for rationality contributes to a number of implicit assumptions about the nature of problems and change. Stacey (2001) uses the phrase 'rationalist teleology' (p. 27) to describe the movement in organisations towards goals and solutions that are reasoned and decided without attention to the less conscious or unspoken dynamics of human experience and interaction, dynamics which, nonetheless, exert a powerful influence on how people feel, think and act.

The dominance of the problem-solution orientation, with its drive for predictability and control, gives rise to a linear and logical approach to root cause analysis and problem solving. This fails to consider constant evolutionary change, the need to be adjusting to complexity in the moment, and the emergent (in the sense of unable to be known in advance) properties of organisations and their participants (Streatfield, 2001). This orientation can find its way into coaching theory and practice where reflection and meaning-making are sacrificed in favour of the pursuit of quick fixes and action.

Watzlavick (2011) has shown that how we approach and formulate problems is key to determining potential resolution. Sometimes the way we frame the problem is a significant part of the problem. As we have discussed earlier, Johnson's (1992) work on polarity management points to the fact that, while certain problems do lend themselves to solutions that can be arrived at through the application of reason and logic, with one obvious solution standing out as the 'right' way relative to other possibilities, many problems in organisations are actually paradoxical in nature, consisting of apparently opposing forces such as reducing costs while maintaining levels of customer service; attending simultaneously to the needs of the individual, team and enterprise; balancing health and safety regulation with commercial and operational pragmatism. These forces, comprising both objective and subjective elements, need to be balanced and kept in some creative tension. Coming down on either side of the dualism will often lead to detrimental impacts. In addition the term 'wicked problem', first coined by West Churchman (1967) has gained in popularity in recent years to describe the complexity of many current challenges such as running the Health Service in the UK, or addressing global warming, where multiple complex factors and polarities make it impossible to know precisely how to act and what the impact of any actions will be. This in turn requires individuals to open to the unknowable, experiment with possibilities, iteratively evaluate impacts and adjust to unintended consequences.

The pursuit of predictability, however, and its function of containing anxiety in the face of 'that which cannot be known in advance', can lead individuals to hold in mind an idea of the solution ahead of any inquiry into the nature of the challenges being faced. This is often based on what one of our client's termed 'yesterday's learning'. This tendency is enshrined in the project management exhortation to 'start with the end in mind'. While it is important to frame intentions regarding the resolution of challenges, where clients are rigidly wedded to a particular solution in mind, they inevitably pre-configure the field of inquiry. They may disregard aspects of their own experience that do not immediately seem relevant to the task in hand. This in turn can constrain the imagination, associative intelligence and bricolage we mentioned in Chapter 5, and the spontaneity necessary for supporting creative adjustments that are more grounded in, and informed by, prevailing field conditions. Heffernan (2011), in her research into the phenomenon of what she terms 'willful blindness', shows how we inevitably discriminate in relation to data by selecting information about a particular situation ... 'that makes us feel great about ourselves, while conveniently filtering whatever unsettles our fragile egos and most vital beliefs' (p. 3). She highlights a whole host of examples to illustrate the disadvantages and devastating consequences of willful blindness including fraud, child abuse and war crimes on a vast scale. For coachees facing complex and ambiguous situations, the pull into selecting data that reassures, and avoiding data that unsettles and calls for deeper reflection, is an understandable temptation, however, Heffernan cautions that the more we leave out, the more powerless we become, calling this the paradox of blindness where we think a belief or practice will make us safe even as it actually is putting us in danger.

Increasingly, the clients we work with report being faced with complex challenges, where different stakeholders and subject-matter experts hold different perspectives and experience different feelings on a given situation. These often need to be aired, and their impact on behaviour examined, in order to break out of entrenched, out of date and unproductive patterns of practice.

The new leader, recently promoted into a more senior role, may struggle with feelings of self-doubt. She may have to manage internal conflicts such as a pressure to be seen to be in control and doing something of value when, in fact, she is still to find her bearings and understand the culture in which she is now working. Similarly, a health and safety manager may find himself needing to manage his own perception of risk and desire to protect others (informed by personal history and feelings of responsibility), while experiencing considerable pressure, hostility, personal criticism and judgement from leaders of commercial departments keen to reduce time consuming and costly safety audits and procedures.

Different perspectives and preoccupations are often taken up and acted out by different individuals in the same organisation. This can fuel conflict, which, in turn, prevents resolution. Many coaching clients bring questions related to how to surface, explore and resolve these differences in service of the organisation's success and well-being. They seem to be becoming aware that it is often the failure to examine the complex field of intersubjectivity and human meaning making and interactions that contributes to, and perpetuates, familiar problems and counterproductive behaviours. Approaches such as Western's network discourse (Western, 2017, 2012), dialogue (Issacs, 1999) and complexity theory (Shaw, 2002) have much to offer coaches and clients in orienting them to taking a wider perspective on a given presenting 'problem'. Laloux (2014) describes that more evolved organisations, which are succeeding in unlocking creativity and innovation, increasingly appreciate and are able to access all domains of knowing. The rational and logical continue to have their uses in these organisations but knowledge is expanded and more holistic. They are able to encompass and access the wisdom in emotion, intuition and even transpersonal psychology, however unsettling this can initially seem relative to the dominant backdrop of organisational rationality and managerial discourse.

Human doing – Human being

Be it supplying produce to supermarkets, caring for the elderly, providing telecommunication services or sending people into outer space, organisations exist to do things. From this emphasis on activities and outputs arises a stance among organisation members that is oriented toward doing and achievement.

On numerous occasions we have had senior leaders comment on feeling disorientated and guilty on moving into more strategic roles where inquiring, reflecting and meaning making are now privileged over doing.

Their new role places particular and personal demands on them. They are required to bring more of themselves to work. They need to be able to slow down, imagine, create and bear confusion and uncertainty (at least temporarily) in order to shape the future and respond flexibly to organisational and environmental changes. Yet, they can still believe they are not contributing. We see this as an illustration of how doing is equated in managerial discourse (Western, 2017, 2012) with a particularly concrete and material idea of contribution, which adds instant, visible, and tangible value. In this context an individual's felt sense of worth is bound up with these assumptions and satisfying the conditions they generate – improve the bottom line, do more, faster and for less! This serves to further illustrate the intimate connection between context and the experience clients have of themselves. In organisations which privilege doing over reflection and meaning making, coaching can provide support for the newly promoted leader who has come from a commercial role into a more strategic role, although we also invite clients to think about what additional support they may need to take up their roles such as joining special interest groups outside of the organisation or communities of practice. Given the intimate relationship between self-experience and context, if we experience little or no support for something that is important to us and necessary for the organisation, we sometimes need to look for that support elsewhere lest we get drawn back into, and be limited by, the dominant orthodoxies of our context.

Bias of individualism in organisational life

One of the consequences of the individualistic bias for many organisations that has a direct bearing on the practice of coaching is the assumption that the individual is the locus of all potency and success. Assessment stresses the individual qualities and developmental needs of the *individual* employee. Successes and failures are thought about primarily in terms of the individual's performance. Some attempts are made to assess employees and put together teams composed of a range of separate styles and attributes, each held by one individual. This still represents a collection of separate entities and does not acknowledge the complex, subtle and dynamic interplay between them. It fails to recognise that self-experience, behaviour and the capacity to think and function are also influenced by the ways in which individuals perceive their organisations, their tasks, each other and their relationships.

An individualist orientation does have its place, however. At times it may be wholly appropriate, and contextually relevant, for a leader to assert an individual perspective or make an authoritative stand. For now we wish to consider those less productive aspects of organisational individualism, and contexts where an unexamined individualist orientation does not support resolution of challenges, learning and development.

Individualism, as we described in the introduction, gives rise to cultures in which thoughts and perspectives are differentiated and reduced often to positions or 'things' in a process known as reification. Here there are right ways and wrong ways of doing things, good and bad answers, acceptable and unacceptable behaviour and 'in' and 'out' crowds depending on different positions held collectively. There can be great individual rewards for perceived successes and much personal shame at failure.

A more relational and contextual perspective would see the individual and his/her attributes as part of a complex field of multiple forces. It is out of the interaction of these forces that perceptions and experiences of success and failure arise. While individuals do learn and grow, the capacity to do so, and the value this learning generates for the organisation are, in large part, determined by how these individuals interact, mutually influence one another, and how this process is either facilitated or impeded by their particular organisational context.

This is a more supportive and realistic paradigm given the complexity of many organisations today. Here projects often depend on the contributions of multiple stakeholders, with authority more distributed than in traditional hierarchies (Hirschhorn, 1997; Laloux, 2014). Drath and Palus (1994) have noted that the nature of many organisational challenges requires different individuals, in different positions in the hierarchy, with different subject matter expertise, biases, assumptions and agendas, to join together to develop shared meaning, intentions, and interventions.

These situations simply do not lend themselves to one leader with all the authority and experience to know what to do to make things happen, and rigid hierarchies where authority is held by those above who are 'served' by those below.

A relational perspective can offer much to coaching clients who, through their implicit individualistic biases, may be assuming more responsibility for outcomes than is realistic or functional. They can be supported in this way to link their personal learning journey to the wider context and the mutual impact between individuals and their environment.

In earlier sections of this book we have set out how polarities and managing polarities is a central component in a relational and integrative orientation to coaching. Laloux (2014) sees this as yet another feature of more evolved organisation cultures. In Chapter 4 we also explored some of the challenges involved in being different or 'other' to the dominant orthodoxies in a given system. We now wish to describe a series of polarities which can be seen to arise in the context of coaching in organisations, which need to be managed, and which face coaches and clients alike with questions related to aligning with or differing from norms.

The following table sets out a number of normative forces which represent one polarity along with those opposite polarities that have less currency in organisations operating from a more traditional set of assumptions and, therefore, can be denied or ignored. The left hand column lists a series of perspectives and patterns of thinking and acting that have come to dominate in many organisations. As a result of their dominance, many organisational difficulties that clients experience can be as a result of an overemphasis on the left hand side, as is the case when one pole of any polarity is overly relied upon (Johnson, 1992). The right hand column represents the opposite polarities to each left hand norm. We have termed these 'emerging patterns' as they often emerge as alternatives to dominant patterns of thinking and acting. They are polarities which may need to be integrated more into how individuals think and act in organisations in order to generate the creativity required to act in timely and effective ways in complex situations, or address seemingly intractable problems, where old thinking and doing more of the same is not having a beneficial impact. Holding the tension of apparently opposite forces is also central to the process of social and psychological bricolage where new strategies can be found through bringing together existing knowledge in new ways.

The different polarities can be thought of as a series of continua describing opposite attitudes and orientations to thinking and acting in organisational life. In order to increase in capacity and creativity for responding to complex organisational and environmental challenges, coaches and coachees need to develop range along each of these continua, balancing the dominant patterns of the left hand column with the new possibilities offered by the emerging pattern on the right. As the range of experience of individuals increases along each continuum, they will be able to choose the orientation and forms of response that are most appropriate to their context and specific moment in time. In situations of relatively low complexity and with few wicked problems, the orientations of the left hand column may be the most functional and appropriate. Development here for coachees may be 'horizontal' where new skills can be acquired, and further assimilated, but where there is no context requirement or desire on the part of the coachee to question the paradigm within which he or she is operating. Moving towards the right hand column involves a shift in paradigm, surfacing and reworking assumptions that might have hitherto been out of conscious

Dominant pattern	Emerging pattern
Objectivity Thought; logic; reason; pre-existing knowledge, meaning and conceptual maps relied upon.	*Subjectivity* Emotion; awareness of perceiving processes; increased awareness of relationship between feelings, thoughts and action; phenomenological orientation; openness to multiple ways of knowing.
Rationalist Teleology Planning; predicting; driving towards pre-determined and tightly defined outcomes; reliance on formulae for change; assumptions about value and success driven from 'expert' or hierarchy; problems seen as all having route causes and ultimately clear solutions. 'It will work here because it worked there'.	*Complexity and Emergence* Attention to tracking and raising awareness of here and now processes of relating and making meaning between individuals; meaning, success and value seen as arising out of dialogue, relating and collaborative inquiry; discrimination brought to problem definition – simple problems differentiated from 'wicked' problems; problems also considered as paradoxical, requiring moment by moment awareness, responsiveness and the resolution of multiple field forces. 'New and complex challenges call for new thinking and acting'.
Doing Attention primarily directed towards activity and actions; privileging of tangible outputs; narrower range of experience and behaviour attended to; reactivity; fast pace.	*Being* Wider range of experience included; action balanced with attention to noticing feelings and thinking processes; presence; deeper listening; reflection; expanded awareness; slower pace.
Individualist paradigm Individual seen as separate and bounded; primary locus of potency, learning and change is situated in the individual; relational stance is one of I-It, subject to object – others seen as objects to be used in service of individual goals.	*Relational, contextual paradigm* Individual experience and 'self' seen as arising from, and being situated in, the environment; self and the process of 'selfing' seen as fluid; potency seen as a function of the dynamic interplay between individual(s) and each environment's dynamics; relational stance of I-Thou, subject to subject – others seen as different subjectivities with whom to explore different meanings and possibilities and consciously establish appropriate and functional levels of consensus; individual and collective success and well-being predicated on collaboration.
Deficit based learning Ideal of some omniscient state; learning designed to plug the gaps; shame at failing to live up to ideals.	*Learning as continuous expansion* Omniscience seen as an illusion and product of egoic identification and striving; learning seen as lifelong and never complete.
Cult of the expert Single individual experts seen as repositories of all relevant knowledge; knowledge transferred down a knowledge/capability gradient from the top to the bottom.	*Varied and distributed expertise* Expertise seen as residing in many individuals; creative possibilities contained in differing perspectives; valuing and supporting the expression of difference not just current orthodoxies or 'expert' opinions; fresh knowledge emerges and is discovered through dialogue and inquiry; knowledge and resolutions created collaboratively.

awareness. This is a feature or 'vertical' development associated with transformational learning (Petrie, 2014, 2015).

Different contexts, different coaches and coachees will demonstrate varying degrees of readiness and openness in relation to vertical development. This will be influenced in large part by their current 'action logic' or developmental stage (Fisher *et al.*, 2003). It is important that as coaches we do not come to this work with an agenda to impose paradigmatic change on clients, even where the field conditions might seem to be calling for it, as this risks being experienced as invasive, coercive and insensitive to the coachee's needs and current capacity for this type of learning. Coaches need to be aware of the challenges in this work and pay attention to balancing the challenge of new thinking with attention to the coachee's and his context's resources and resilience for engaging with ways of thinking that may be radical and unsettling relative to what is familiar to them. Coaches also need to be aware of their own action logic and how this guides their own meaning making and action with their clients. There are now a number of measurement tools which can accurately assess an individual's current stage of development. These not only provide coaches and coachees with a sense of their current stage of development, but also can provide guidance and support to enable ongoing vertical development where this might be desired. Even where vertical development objectives are clearly articulated, for example as part of a strategic leadership development programme, it is not possible to know how coachees will respond to deep questioning of long held assumptions, established norms and familiar approaches. The very nature of transformational learning is such that we cannot know if we actually want what we are aiming for until we experience it. We might like the idea of being able to navigate multiple perspectives on an issue and creatively respond to complexity from a place of emotional, intuitive and cognitive knowing, only to discover that the unsettling that this development inevitably brings with it leads us, under pressure, to revert to anxiety based control mechanisms and past strategies.

We find it useful in working in this way to draw upon the metaphor of hinting we described in Chapter 8. In the reciprocal dance of the coaching conversation coachees will be offering 'hints' about their ways of seeing the world and readiness for vertical development. As we said earlier, in a relational orientation to coaching, the coach's use of self as a catalytic 'other' who can introduce novelty and different perspectives into the conversation is key to facilitating change. The coach may offer a number of 'hints' at the possibility of seeing things differently in the form of a question or 'thinking aloud' with the coachee. In this way the coach can continue to track what the coachee is making for himself of the coach's gestures into the conversation and, together with the coachee, evaluate the extent to which these are in service of the coachee's learning and development in ways appropriate to the context.

We now turn our attention to ways in which the dominant norms can find their way into the coaching conversation and how coaches might 'hint' at other possibilities.

Dynamics arising in the coaching relationship

A relational approach to coaching offers an orientation which allows for inquiry into the dynamics of the coaching relationship, and the moment by moment unfolding of client and coach experience, in service of awareness, change and development. As we have described at various points, clients often bring and embody the dominant patterns and norms of their context into the relationship with their coach. Furthermore, the coaching relationship, occurring as it does in the context of an organisational field, can also offer up data about the impact of that field on both client and coach, as well as a container in which to explore these impacts and expand range and choice for responding.

Working to expand coachee range

As we have set out, relationally oriented practice sees the individual and field mutually influencing each other. Thus a change in one can bring about a change in the other, and vice versa. Many approaches to coaching in the current literature are themselves infused with similar assumptions to those that underpin a number of the dominant norms we have been discussing. Sequential stage models, process maps, pre-determined outcome orientation, all can dominate, to the extent that the rich territory of relatedness is less explored and under-utilised in the service of client and organisational growth.

This is not to imply that specific methodologies, coaching contracts and intended outcomes, which are lightly held, do not have their place. In many ways they are necessary for earning credibility in the organisational domain and for bounding and focusing the work. What we are suggesting is that, with a relational orientation, the coach's presence, and personal relationship to the qualities of the emerging patterns described in the table above, are what can contribute to creating a sufficiently novel force or difference to support deeper reflection, meaning making and expansion of client repertoires for responding. If the coaching conversation can become a generative conversation expanding the mindset of coachees it stands to influence and change conversations out in the wider organisation.

We now wish to outline some of the ways in which the dominant norms and patterns of thought can reveal themselves in the coaching relationship, the responses they can give rise to in coaches, and ways in which coaches might begin to experiment with allowing the emergent into their work and client interactions.

The following descriptions are drawn from our experience with coachees, students and supervisees. We give examples of how a particular dominant way of thinking or being can manifest in the coaching relationship and conversation. We describe some of the 'resonances' (as described in Chapter 8) a coach may experience, which are ways in which we pick up hints about the coachee's inner world and dominant paradigm. We then describe a number of ways in which the coach might articulate these resonances in the form of a thought or behaviour to create a novel force for coachees to engage with. Where these can be picked up and made use of, they stand to support movement towards the more emerging pattern end of the continuum. Wherever we offer suggestions for moving towards an integration of the emerging pattern all the pointers we discussed in Chapter 8 about the coach being a source of difference apply.

As is the case with all examples, these are not presented here as an exhaustive list, nor as definitive. It is inevitable that dominant patterns will reveal themselves in a multitude of different ways, and as coaches we will equally be impacted in a host of ways based on our own development level, patterning, preferences and the degree of reflexivity and experimentation we experience as possible in each unique coach-coachee-context situation. Each of the following examples also describes some of the ways in which coach and coachee mutually influence one another.

Objectivity – Subjectivity

Manifestation of dominant pattern

Here the client might demonstrate a particular way of thinking about his role and developmental challenges characterised by generalised assumptions and beliefs about himself and the world. He will want a coach who can demonstrate (often in advance) logically and rationally what he needs to do in order to be successful. Reliance on prior knowledge and a tendency towards reduction dominate. There will be little tolerance of ambiguity and nuance. The potential for new insights and perspectives to arise is limited, as the content of conversation tends to lean towards what is already known, familiar and safe. Access to feeling and embodied experience will be restricted.

Resonances in the coach

As the coach you may feel a need to keep justifying why you work the way you do. You may experience, or imagine, that unless you make explicit every step of your thinking and rationale, you will not be understood, or will be dismissed by the client. You may find your own thought processes becoming superficial, mechanistic and formulaic. Relational contact will be low.

Orienting to the emerging pattern

Resist the pull to give a rationale for every thought and intervention. You might disclose reactions and thoughts and check to see whether they resonate with the client and, if so, how. If interventions do not make instant rational sense to the client, you may wish to invite him to report on his responses to what you have just said (even if he feels or understands little). Adopt a stance that is allowing and acknowledging of your own feelings. Track the client's process of being with you and the use he might be making of your interventions, and be willing to drop them if you feel you are losing the client's attention. You might invite the client to pay attention to how he is feeling in relation to his challenges, you, and the way you are working. Offer a matter of fact consideration of the role of feelings in organisational life. Be prepared to use examples or make educative interventions to help bridge the mind-body split.

Rationalist teleology – Complexity and emergence

Manifestation of the dominant pattern

The client will be primarily oriented towards processes and methodologies for change. She may demonstrate a high need for predictability and pre-determined outcomes. She is likely to be uncomfortable with contingency, the unpredictable and emergent. Lacking support to hold a more complex view of the underlying dynamics in herself, others, or in her organisation, she may retreat into rigid structures and processes. This can serve to contain anxiety and create the illusion of mastery over the unpredictable. Thinking 'out of the box' will be difficult.

Resonances in the coach

Unless you share the client's bias for control and containment of the unpredictable, you might feel constrained and contracted in your range of feeling and thinking. Any strong sensations and intuitive insights might feel risky and problematic. This is as a result of there being little room in the co-created relational field (co-transference) to play with possibilities, form tentative hypotheses and test them out. You may find yourself disregarding thoughts, images and associations that do not fit within a tightly structured logical sequence of ideas. You may feel that the conversation is 'surface' rather than deep.

Orienting to the emerging pattern

Ground yourself in a phenomenological stance and practice horizontalising, where you treat everything that happens in the client, in you, the relationship and wider context as potentially relevant. You might name what you see and feel, and check for resonance with the coachee. Be prepared for the fact that many of your interventions may initially fall very flat. Watch any pull to make instant impact! Remember coachees may take time to consider observations and possibilities that take them outside of familiar territory. Over time the coachee may come to see that aspects of the field and wider context, which made little sense in the past, now seem to be relevant. Track meaning making processes in the coachee and in yourself, and resist the temptation to quickly make observations fit into pre-existing conceptual maps. Hold meaning lightly and practice openness to updating it in light of new data and insights.

Doing – Being

Manifestation of the dominant pattern

The coachee will come expecting action. He may display low tolerance of inquiry and relationship building. He may want to know exactly how coaching can help him behave differently ahead of any inquiry or contracting. He may implicitly see the coach as an extension of the organisation's hierarchy and expect to be told what to do in order to succeed in the system.

Resonances in the coach

You can feel under pressure to make things happen fast. You may find yourself working hard to come up with elaborate action plans on the coachee's behalf. You can feel under pressure to suggest solutions, rather than take the time to inquire with the client and explore the organisational field and the client's relationship to it. Meaning making can be rapidly inferential. You may feel your capacity to surface underlying field conditions to be limited or unavailable. There may be a pressured and agitated quality to interactions with the client.

Orienting to the emerging pattern

Slow down and take time to sense into yourself. Hold back on making solution-oriented interventions, resist the pull to get busy. Pay attention to self-support, presence, breathing and grounding. Work at being a more reflective presence. Be willing to articulate the emotional/energetic field for what it might reveal of the organisation and your and your client's relationship to it. Spend time inquiring into field conditions. Acknowledge any discomfort in the client.

Individualistic paradigm – Relational and contextual paradigm

Manifestation of the dominant pattern

The coachee will tend to consider herself to be the centre of all learning and change. She will look to developing her range and repertoire in the belief that this is the only way to make a difference. She may move between the positions of omnipotence and impotence. She may downplay or ignore the field conditions in which she works, or the other relationships that are also critical to making things happen. A common orienting belief is 'if only *I* were more/less . . .

I could do . . .'. The relational stance of the coachee towards others is I-It (Buber, 1958) or 'subject-object' where others are seen as needing to be influenced in service of the individual's agenda.

Resonances in the coach

As coach, you too may find yourself focusing on the coachee to the exclusion of the wider field and its impact on her experience of herself and her challenges. The work will tend to move in the direction of looking primarily at the coachee as if she were a closed system isolated from context. You may find that you are paying little or no attention to your relationship with the coachee and the subtleties of mutual influence, suggestive of actually being caught in a particular co-created phenomenon!

Orienting to the emerging pattern

Remember, whatever you are working on with coachees that is pertinent to their personality characteristics and individual learning contracts, the work is taking place in a system of relationships. Coachees' thoughts and feelings reveal not only their inner processing and meaning making, but will contain data about how they are being impacted consciously and unconsciously by the environment in which they work. Remind coachees of the dynamic interplay between their experience and perceptions and those of others. You can model this by drawing attention to the way you and your coachee mutually influence each other in the coaching relationship.

Deficit model of learning – Learning as continuous unfolding

Manifestation of the dominant pattern

The coachee who holds a belief that learning is focused on dealing with deficits is likely to be less supported in herself and prone to shame. She may see coaching as remedial rather than supportive and developmental. There may be some truth in this, where a subtext to coaching might be to bring a client in line with behavioural expectations and ideals held by senior members of the organisation hierarchy. The client with this pattern of self-organisation may look to the coach to tell her what to think and do. She may feel or believe she has little experience and knowledge to draw upon.

Resonances in the coach

You may feel you have to tread carefully if you are resonating with any fragility in the client. Alternatively, you may unconsciously pick up on the client's desire to be told what to do, and find yourself getting busy and working hard on the client's behalf.

Orienting to the emerging pattern

Be interested in the coachee's experience and views. Hold back on getting busy. Instead, ask the coachee for her thoughts and perspectives and respond in ways that communicate your interest and willingness to understand. Work to surface what resources the coachee can draw upon in herself. You can also ask the coachee what interests her and co-create a learning contract that balances organisation requirements with the coachee's own areas of concern.

Cult of the expert – Varied and distributed expertise

Manifestation of the dominant pattern

The coachee can project 'expert' onto the coach. He may appear to hang on the coach's every word. It is also possible that the coachee will feel diminished by his own projection and disowning of his capabilities, appearing ambivalent towards you and your interventions. The coachee may appear not to trust his own thinking and look to you to validate this. He may become dependent on you (and vice versa!), telephoning frequently in order to run his thinking by you ahead of any meeting or intervention.

Resonances in the coach

The conversation can feel one-sided. You may find yourself talking a lot and working hard. If you have concerns about your own competence you may feel shored up by the coachee's apparent interest and willingness to accord you regard and status, or anxious that, at any moment now, you could let him down given the weight of expectation upon you, or be exposed as an impostor.

Orienting to the emerging pattern

Be prepared to disclose your own uncertainties and confusion. Demonstrate your comfort with not knowing or not being sure, and your capacity to think things through with the coachee. Model reflective practice in order that the coachee can learn how to do this for himself and connect with his own resources, rather than imagine you, the coach, have all the answers. Where a coachee is ambivalent about the power he has accorded you, it can be useful to be willing to bumble a little, being human rather than superhuman or overly polished. Resist any pull to 'tell' or impart wisdom.

In the examples above we hope to have illustrated some of the ways in which the coach, coachee and context interact to give rise to particular feelings, thoughts and behaviours. It is by holding this dynamic interplay in mind that relationally oriented coaches can extend their range for working more holistically in service of individual and organisational learning and change.

Author note

Many of the perspectives in this chapter first appeared in Cavicchia, S. (2009) 'Towards a relational approach to coaching – Integrating the disavowed aspects', *International Gestalt Journal*, 32 (1), 49–80.

Chapter 12

Feedback and assessment

In this chapter we wish to examine the ways in which feedback has come to be constructed and thought about in organisations and the ways in which individualism and the notion of an objective observer permeate the ways in which data are gathered, made use of and communicated. We shall consider what a situational, relational and intersubjective orientation might have to offer coaches and their clients in terms of how feedback is understood, thought about and used in service of individual and organisational development.

The Newtonian organisation – Individualism, positivism and the 'official' uses of feedback

Feedback in organisational life is considered to be a fundamental mechanism for enabling people to understand themselves, learn and develop. Feedback is seen to be a process whereby individuals can obtain information about how they are perceived and how they are performing against their organisation's criteria for, and working assumptions about, what is required to be individually and collectively successful. Feedback is often closely connected to competency and behaviour frameworks, the particular constructs that reflect an organisation's current thinking and ideology about what makes for an effective and desirable employee – a good 'corporate citizen'.

This common construction of feedback inevitably reflects to some extent the mechanistic and positivist perspectives on organisation and human 'systems', which include viewing organisations and their members as separate entities that can be observed, measured and broken down into constituent parts. As we set out in previous chapters, with these approaches there is an implicit leaning towards Cartesian duality, predictability, control and a mechanistic bias for linear thinking and cause and effect logic (Gergen, 2009). Many psychometric tests are steeped in this tradition and look for recurring and measurable individual traits, behaviour patterns and thinking styles that then might be used to predict suitability for role, potential success, and fit with a particular job description or function. They also identify areas for individual development necessary to bring individuals in line with organisational and role expectations.

This particular viewing angle, while offering one way of shaping, perceiving and thinking about organisations and the people who come together to form them, can also distance people from one another, reducing them to phenomena that can be observed and manipulated. It risks simplification and objectifying of the uniqueness of individuals and the subtle complexities of their situated experience, subjectivity and interactions as organisation participants. These subtle variables, which may not always be observable at the surface of clichéd and enculturated behaviours, mission statements, formulaic processes and personality classifications, nonetheless, exert a potent influence on what actually happens in organisations – how the people who form them feel, experience themselves, make meaning, learn, perform and change.

Patterns of thought and behaviour (culture) have developed around the uses of feedback which reflect these positivist biases and the perceived importance of feedback along with the meanings with which it is invested. We have worked in a number of organisations that extoll the virtues of feedback with posters stating: 'Feedback is a gift! Do not get defensive! Always thank the giver!'. These, and similar exhortations, can serve to create a set of rules (based on sound principle) designed to support a particular engagement with feedback and yet, as the direct experience of many of our clients suggests, can be experienced as clichéd and superficial ways of interacting in relation to a process that is far from straightforward – an attempt to logically and 'rationally' facilitate an exchange that can often be *experienced* as anxiety provoking, complex, ambiguous, multi-layered, unsettling, subjective, challenging and not always 'helpful'. Rules and exhortations related to the 'correct' way to engage with feedback exert pressure on individuals to split off and drive underground any responses which do not align with surface expectations, potentially reinforcing a false self-real self split where individuals act out a role rather than bring more of their difference and uniqueness to the organisation where this may be necessary and desirable for effective functioning.

Within the positivist tradition which privileges logic and reason, the giving and receiving of feedback can come to be seen as a transactional process which, if skillfully executed, will result in beneficial and predictable impacts. Many of our clients, as well as students and supervisees, can become caught in a tyranny of perfection around ensuring that the messages they deliver are so finely honed that they can only be heard in a useful and 'appropriately developmental' way by the recipient. This is not a particularly helpful assumption when dealing with human beings, personality structure and subjectivity. Nor is it useful when encountering ambiguity, complex and shifting organisation contexts, along with inevitable preoccupations with questions of performance, value, security, self worth, belonging and identity. Although it is important to think about how best to deliver feedback in a way that enables the giver to be authentic, while respecting the integrity of the recipient, it is never possible to know in advance how feedback will be heard and made use of. Instrumental approaches to feedback, coaching and consulting can drive an obsession with 'getting the message right to get the impact right', where 'right' often means alignment with organisational expectations for an individual.

This in turn fuels training approaches that concentrate on acquiring feedback 'skills'. There is a focus on the stance and language of the giver, reflecting linear and mechanistic assumptions about communication as a process of transmission as opposed to a dance of mutual and reciprocal meaning making and negotiation of different perspectives. Tools and stage models can provide a degree of structure to contain anxiety and guide individuals through the subtle and complex territory of human intersubjectivity, but can also fail to appreciate the nature and dynamics of these interactions. If they are over-relied on, coaches risk becoming overly instrumental and fail to develop the attunement and sensitivity required for tracking the relational processes that occur between people in the act of attempting to make meaning together about themselves, their organisations and their place within them.

To a great extent, much of this is inevitable. Organisations do need to define themselves, place boundaries around what they currently are and are not, and construct narratives in relation to what they do and how they work. As environments, organisations cannot but make demands on their members that call on them to hold a tension between individual desires and preferences and organisational and role requirements (Gantt and Agazarian, 2005; Western, 2017, 2012) (See Chapter 4). This gives rise to a number of features characteristic of feedback in an organisational context reflecting the more traditional/positivist biases. While they may not all be present or visible in all organisations, they can be seen in many.

Tightly prescribed parameters (of acceptability, of perceptual frames and meaning making)

Given the tendency to tie feedback in with performance, capability and behavioural criteria, parameters are established which demarcate the territory of what can be noticed, observed and commented upon. This can result in the premature foreclosure of meaning and missed opportunities for individual and collective learning. An emotional outburst by a leader in an organisation which privileges calm and polite formality, might be viewed through a lens of 'inappropriate' behaviour, and the leader forever labeled as volatile and problematic. In this way opportunities are missed for deeper inquiry into what was behind the outburst, what other factors of the leader's and organisation's current situation might be giving rise to this particular behavioural phenomenon, and whether emotion and passion might just have something to offer in revitalising conversation and creativity. The same could be said of an attitude of calm reflexivity in a competitive and highly energetic sales environment being interpreted as lacking in drive and 'hunger' for results, even where the latter is resulting in inappropriate and catastrophic decision making as was the case with the global financial crisis (Financial Crisis Inquiry Report, 2011).

There is often, appropriately, a tendency toward naming observable phenomena and hard facts (even though what is noticed or stands out for people is already, in part, determined by the particulars of a specific organisation's culture and the perceptual preferences this gives rise to). However, there can be less conscious attention paid to the way meaning is inferred and derived from these facts, especially the interplay of emotion, affect and cognition (Cozolino, 2006; Damasio, 2000). Given the fast pace of much organisational life, there is often little time made to slow down and examine assumptions and meaning making processes, or increase the angles from which a particular phenomenon might be viewed. This can give rise to partial or distorted perspectives on individuals akin to those brought about by the distorted glass in a fair ground hall of mirrors. Partial and distorted perspectives which nonetheless can become fixed in the minds of others and impact the quality of relating and interaction.

As we described earlier, we have often been asked to coach individuals who are seen to be 'problematic' in some way, usually meaning that something about them differs from the dominant and 'official' orthodoxies governing behaviour in a particular organisation. Where they have agreed to work with us, we are frequently delighted and surprised to find that our experience of them is not always that of those who might have commissioned the work. While a relational view of the self as a dynamic process which is impacted by, and shaped in, different contexts explains how this can arise, this is still a challenging situation to be in. As coaches we need to guard against over privileging the particular version of the client we are experiencing, while also holding this as being of equal value and potential relevance to the version of the client as experienced by, and co-constructed, with stakeholders and customers. Holding both versions allows for exploration of how these differences in experience, behaviour and perception might have come about in the different contexts of the organisation and coaching relationship. This can support the process of bricolage where coachees might be supported to consider how they might transfer positive and appropriate elements of their way of being from one setting into another, and can guard against the coach becoming an instrument of social control and manipulation.

Hierarchy and power

In organisational contexts, which are often hierarchical, where those above are able to wield actual or perceived power and authority over those below, rapid, premature and partial meaning making about an individual's personality and performance can become highly charged. Once a senior leader has formed a particular opinion of an individual (good or bad) to which he/she is very wedded, it is likely to become hard for others to question or expand upon it. Once fixed in this way, it can be exceedingly difficult for the individual who has been assigned a role, or been 'typecast', to become anything else in the eyes of others. This represents a challenge to the individualistic notion embedded in much coaching theory that all agency for change resides within the person of the client.

More often (as we explored in Chapter 10) than might be acknowledged, it is the forces at work in the system, including the perceptions individuals have of one another, which determine an individual's capacity for change, at least as much as, and at times more than, any individually located capacity, agency or motivation.

Belonging and 'boundary policing' (to monitor whether you fit in or not)

Given the close relationship in organisations between feedback and what the organisation considers to be a 'good' corporate citizen, it inevitably comes to represent a mechanism whereby individuals get to see the extent to which they are perceived to be complying or not with what is desired, and performing within acceptable parameters. This in turn gives rise to anxiety and goes some way to explaining why 'negative' or 'developmental' feedback can be so distressing for clients (and coaches!). For not only are they potentially faced with new information which needs to be deconstructed, adjusted to, and their self images/personality unsettled and updated accordingly, but also shame based anxiety related to fear of rejection or exclusion is frequently activated, along with survival fears associated with perceived reputational damage. Given these concerns, a situation arises where feedback can subtly and not so subtly become a mechanism for persona manipulation, driving homogeneity and compliance. However much organisations might talk of valuing difference, over the years we have been struck by how difficult it can be for individuals in organisations to consider and contemplate differences for what they might have to offer, even when 'doing more of the same' is clearly failing to deliver the necessary or desired results.

We are not suggesting that compliance with patterns of behaviour and the achievement of prescribed targets set within the organisation environment are a bad thing. Far from it. These often provide narrative and enduring identity along with other necessary structures and constraints to bound the field of activity and focus limited resources in specific and productive ways. At the individual level, understanding the requirements of context and adjusting appropriately constitute the fundamental process of taking up a role. However, the complexity of many organisations and the challenges they and their employees face, along with the need to generate new patterns and levels of flexibility and responsiveness in the face of shifting internal and external environments, require that their members also be able to consider differences and divergence from norms and integrate these where appropriate as we explored in the previous chapter. Where feedback is used primarily to drive compliance, opportunities can be missed for necessary creativity and generativity. Neurotic anxiety associated with fear of losing control or position comes to dominate thinking and acting. This often results in frenetic activity to the extent that organisation participants never learn to bear the existential anxiety necessary for facing the unknown and consciously creating new meanings, new versions of self and, potentially, more productive behavioural strategies and organisational forms.

In thinking about feedback in the context of coaching and consulting in organisations, a relational perspective emphasises that the phenomenon of feedback cannot but be influenced by the context, time and situation in which it is happening. We have so far considered aspects of the ways in which feedback is made use of more consciously and 'officially'. We now wish to explore the multitude of 'unofficial' interactions that also contribute to the dynamics of feedback in organisational life.

Quantum organising – Towards a complex, situational and relational view of feedback – Surfacing the 'unofficial'

As we have described, organisations are increasingly coming to be viewed as contexts of human interaction where meanings, behaviours and organisation itself (as patterns of interaction, processes and their impacts) arise out of the complex moment-by-moment interactions of their members who can be thought of as participating in the 'organising' of the enterprise. It is these interactions that can be thought about as feedback loops which, in addition to the official forms feedback can take, are unofficial in that they do not constitute formal or necessarily conscious mechanisms for generating meaning about individuals, their organisation and their relationship to it. Yet they are *fundamental* in this process. Individual gestures (conversations, instructions, requests, reactions, facial expressions, tones of voice, levels of energetic expression, relational connections/ruptures and so on) are made meaning of with varying degrees of conscious awareness, and then responded to on the basis of these meanings which, in turn, give rise to new gestures and so on. From a relational and interactional perspective, these gestures and responses could even be considered to underpin *all* organisational patterning of which formal and official uses of feedback are simply one particular enduring pattern or construction.

In organisation terms, the process of 'selfing' (how an individual organises his or her feelings, thinking and action into an experiential sense of self moment by moment (see Chapter 2)) that is enacted in and through the medium of unofficial feedback loops constitutes the process of organising individually and collectively. This, in turn, gives rise to and maintains the moment-by-moment apparent forms organisations take, which shape intentions, behaviours, activities and patterns of interaction. A particular repetitive 'patterning' can persist over time, giving the impression of stability and structure. This can lead individuals to play down, or miss altogether, the interactive processes that, through repetition, are what maintain certain apparently enduring patterns in place. If these were to be changed, then new patterns could emerge.

While we are often involved with clients in exploring feedback obtained through official processes and more positivist methodologies, we are equally, if not more, involved in helping clients make sense of their subjective experience of the myriad of interactions they participate in on a daily basis with superiors, peers, direct reports, customers and suppliers, and which represent environmental stimuli, gestures and responses that inevitably impact their process of creative adjustment to daily challenges, self-experience and individual and collective behaviour. The coaching relationship offers a space in which these dynamics can be thought about and new strategies for interacting developed, which then can inform and stand to change interactions in the wider organisational field.

The client who, in spite of setting out clear objectives for his new team, finds that team members rarely follow through on their stated commitments and are surly and disengaged in meetings; the client whose boss persists in publicly criticising her; the client who has to find ways to engage different stakeholders in a matrix organisation in service of his own business success, where he has no positional authority to make things happen, and stakeholders are angrily telling him they are currently too busy to help; the client who experiences a feeling of inadequacy whenever her manager looks at her 'funny' – these are but a few typical examples of the multitude of situations we are involved in making sense of with clients in order to support their capacity to respond in increasingly creative, timely and effective ways, balancing attention to individual vulnerabilities, needs and preferences with the requirements of the environment. This involves exploring, negotiating and constructing meaning from the different perspectives of the client, coach and others in the field.

Clients inevitably bring their experiences of the organisation into the coaching relationship and conversation. It seems to us that making sense of these experiences can be an important part of coaching intended to support creative, reflective and responsive behaviours in coachees, which, in turn, stand to influence the patterns of interaction that shape organisations and the experiences of their people and vice versa.

Feedback and feedback loops as both explicit or implicit information, formal or informal, official or unofficial, conscious or unconscious communication, are central to how individuals experience themselves moment by moment in organisations and everyday life which, in turn, informs how they organise and act. If we hold with this proposition, then development and change for individuals and organisations (given that from a relational perspective the two are indivisible) is a function of the ways in which individuals might be supported to engage with this interplay more consciously in order to increase behavioural options and support greater awareness and choice in how to respond and engage with one another.

Coaching practice considerations – Re-working individual and collective organising

In Chapter 4 we explored in some detail the relationship between individual self-experience and organisation dynamics. We revisit some of the ideas explored there in the context of working relationally with feedback.

Attention to meaning making processes and facilitating 'contact' with feedback

Working with clients to enable them to make sense of feedback potentially affords them the opportunity to learn about themselves; consider the perceptions of others; choose to take on or reject aspects of the feedback; learn about their context, the perceptual frames and preoccupations of feedback givers and other stakeholders; explore their own meaning making processes and experiment with new possibilities; choose how they wish to adjust to feedback (and their organisational context); and ultimately explore consequences of options before committing to a course of action (which may include aware and chosen inaction). A relational intersubjective orientation is particularly suited to a project of this kind. It involves shifting a focus from taking things at face value and identifying with information and meanings arising out of formal and informal feedback interactions, to attending to the process of meaning-making itself, acknowledging the more dynamic aspects of self-experience.

Gestalt (Wheeler, 2000) offers a detailed framework for observing how individuals make contact with the environment. Known as modifications to contact (Joyce and Sills, 2014), they provide an extremely useful frame for exploring how clients relate to the environment, feedback and their experience of, and participation in, organisational interactions. Clients benefit enormously in the coaching relationship from being offered the possibility to hold information, feedback and their meaning-making lightly, slowing down the at times reflex tendency to either introject (swallow whole), particularly if prone to merger with the organisation and anxiety about fitting in, or reject, if inclined towards separateness and anxiety about being overwhelmed and losing a sense of self.

Tracking and bringing to awareness a particular client's ways of making contact with and assimilating feedback and data from the environment goes to the heart of an individual's selfing process in their particular work context. Feedback can evoke historical patterns of self-organisation, particularly in superior-subordinate interactions. By surfacing these patterns in the here and now, clients can be supported to see they have more choice in how they respond to their superiors than they might have if they approach these interactions from a self-organisation of 'child' to their superior as imagined 'critical parent'.

Attention to authority dynamics and their impact

With formal and informal feedback, the particular position in the organisation hierarchy of those giving feedback, and their actual or perceived power to influence the future of the recipients, will have a bearing on the way feedback is given, made use of, and interactions made sense of. Furthermore, clients may need to explore their relationship to the way in which particular patterns of thinking and behaviour have become established in their organisation and sanctioned by those in authority. It can be useful to explore whether a client may be needing or wanting to comply with, or might need or want to appropriately question, authority in the service of learning, individual and organisational well-being and success. Does their role and the nature of their challenges call for more risking of self in challenging orthodoxies that might actually be detrimental to the organisation's effectiveness and productivity? A senior leader used her coaching to explore and become clear that she believed it important to tackle a series of legacy issues that were proving to be problematic, expensive and impractical. This was in spite of the fact that the cultural tendency in the organisation was to not rock the boat and where, in spite of a public narrative supporting change, there was much private emotional attachment to maintaining the status quo among senior leaders.

Attention to support

Formal and informal feedback interactions in organisations can be experienced as unsettling and destabilising. Primarily this hinges on the centrality of relational connection to others for our sense of well-being and continuity, which is intensified in organisational life by anxiety about membership, personal and professional security and the implicit individualism at the heart of most organisation cultures. Here the opinion of others can have real, material and serious consequences for an individual's reputation and future. The individualistic biases of many organisations mean that the field is rarely supportive of a meaningful engagement with feedback. Too much is often literally, or imagined to be, at stake, where heroes one day can become zeros the next.

Gestalt psychology has made a significant contribution to understanding the intimate relationship between the qualities and nature of support in the field and the experience of support, coherence and agency in individuals (Lee and Wheeler, 1996). While some organisations offer conditions in which to relate, collaborate and create, truly valuing difference and enabling the fulfillment of personal, professional and collective potential, this is relatively rare (Laloux, 2014). Forces for control, while offering definition, can also fuel neurotic anxiety and an, at times, unhealthy and limiting preoccupation with fitting in.

All of these factors contribute to increasing the sensitivity of coachees to how they might be being constructed in the minds of others. This is particularly present where they perceive that they are being misrepresented or misconstrued relative to their intentions, how they see themselves, how they might wish to be seen, and how they believe they might need to be seen in order to remain secure and productive in their contexts.

Relational coaching can support clients to take a more context-aware perspective on feedback, alerting them to the co-constructed nature of feedback and relational interactions, and supporting them to inquire into how it might be that they are being constructed in particular ways in the minds of others, the part they might be playing in this, and what the construction might also be saying about the preoccupations and concerns of their colleagues. Widening the viewing angle in this way can support clients to regain a sense of reflective engagement with feedback and can support taking greater responsibility for their own part in the co-construction than if they become mired in defensive rejection of experiences and feedback data which feel too alien, punishing or threatening to engage with. Imagining and understanding the perceptual frames of feedback givers can also yield information that clients can make use of to experiment with different patterns of relating more likely to meet others in a climate of appreciation, understanding and collaboration.

It is important to mention aggression here as part of the support clients may need. The pressure to conform can be so great that clients frequently retroflect (turn inwards) feelings of aggression or disgust (Philippson, 2012) in the face of exchanges and feedback they feel misrepresented or hurt by in some way. They may believe they need to be seen to 'take it on the chin', or that any sign of vulnerability will be seen as implying weakness or unprofessionalism. It is a normal human reaction to feel angry or distressed if we believe we have been misconstrued. If this is retroflected, anger at the environment becomes anger at self where it then fuels self-doubt and inner self-criticism.

Perls's (1951) view that aggression, as life force, supports discernment, knowing what is right and good for us and a healthy engagement with living is potentially useful for coaches in the context of feedback. It can act as an antidote to swallowing whole feedback and internalising interactions that might be inappropriate, overly critical or shaming in some way. Aggression in this sense supports greater discrimination and reflection on feedback. The coach has a potential role in supporting the coachee to temper both wholesale introjection and rejection so that she might see how she is making meaning from feedback or interactions that she cannot fully understand, or which trigger her in some way that leaves her lacking in resilience, support and feeling defensive.

If coachees feel misconstrued, as coaches we often only have their version of events. We need to guard against taking sides either with the giver of feedback or with the coachee, and instead support clients to look at the meaning that is being made and what choices they have for influencing the relational dance with colleagues and stakeholders that might result in a more accurate assessment of their contribution/potential, or different interactional pattern that is more supportive to individual and organisational well-being and success.

It can be important initially to make space for clients to experience the discomfort and anger they might be feeling as the result of an interaction or formal piece of feedback. This offers an experience of confirmation, where their experience is taken seriously and attuned to by the coach. This can give rise to a profound experience of acceptance in coachees, which contrasts with the familiar lack of acknowledgement of feelings and individual subjectivity in much organisational life. A number of our clients over the years have presented as energetically flat and hopeless in the face of these exchanges, often revealing a vicious inner critic fuelled by their own disowned and retroflected aggression. If these clients can be supported to acknowledge their anger at the other or the situation they find themselves in, they stand to reconnect with healthy and appropriate aggression in service of discrimination and reflection in the face of what they have experienced.

A client had for years experienced her line manager as abrasive and bullying. This had resulted in her withdrawing further and further from the relationship and her own inner resources. She had lost a wider perspective and started to doubt herself and her capacities. She was able to make use of her coach to discover and feel into her burning desire to scream at her boss and tell him how angry his treatment of her, as she saw it, made her feel. As she felt the energy, strength and solidity this acknowledgement gave rise to in her body, she was able to reconnect with a sense of capacity and agency. She then became more able to reflect on and evaluate options, she clearly saw the potential risk and inappropriateness in confronting her boss as directly as part of her might have wished to. Instead, she found a way to use her newly discovered clarity, strength and resilience, as a result of reclaiming her legitimate feelings, to contribute more to meetings and conversations with her line manager. This resulted in his becoming more interested in what she had to say and a reduction in his comments and exchanges that she had experienced as passive aggression. In her appraisal he commented that he had really noticed her contributing more and that he valued this, having been frustrated by her withdrawal, which he had construed as her being disinterested and disconnected. Through experiencing the support of her appropriate aggression, and being willing to experiment with a new relational move, this client was able to bring about a different and more generative pattern of interaction with her line manager and engage more fully with her work.

Mindfulness and somatic practices designed to increase connection with sensation and contain impulses to act out in inappropriate ways can be particularly useful here in supporting clients to manage their emotional arousal and increase reflection and choice. Feelings then become a source of information about what is going on for a client in a particular situation rather than simply being impulses to be feared or acted upon. Furthermore, as we described in earlier chapters, increased somatic connection can confer a sense of deeper connection to self and a sense of self beyond mental content and preoccupations with self-image.

A relational perspective offers a way of understanding the experience of constructing, communicating and receiving feedback and the wider contextual dynamics that are at play. It stands to cut across the tendency to either swallow whole or reject meanings outright. Surfacing more of the total situation in which feedback and feedback loops arise for what it might have to offer in terms of meaning making can support a more reflective engagement with feedback, creative adjustment and responsiveness in our clients. Holding feedback conversations and supporting clients to make sense of both official and unofficial feedback experiences is an area where a relational orientation has much to offer coachees and their organisations.

A contextual, relational approach to sense making from feedback cannot simply be solely about coaching someone into alignment with organisational expectations, which would take on dangerous connotations of coaching being used as an instrument for social control. Nor is it about purely coaching an individual in relation to their personal objectives as if isolated from context. Rather it is a process of supporting the client to engage with, deconstruct, assimilate and adjust to the feedback (in every sense) they are experiencing, which includes the holding of personal preferences, versions of self and objectives alongside those of the organisation and stakeholders with whom the individual has to interact. This often involves exploring possible consequences of alignment with (sameness) and separation from (difference) the dominant patterns of the organisation and its participants. If a client can feel supported in the face of imagined consequences, and come to trust they can adjust to the as yet unknowable, then there will be support in both directions. This is a particularly important line of inquiry in contexts of increased uncertainty and complexity where there are no clear right or wrong positions, but where choosing from among a range of options for action and experimenting might be required in order to discover what might actually work in practice.

Concluding thoughts

Relational perspectives on the development of coaches, ethics and supervision

In keeping with the emphasis and focus of this book, we wish to end by pointing to a number of implications of an integrative and relational orientation for the development of coaches, for ethical considerations and for supervision. The approach we have set out privileges the interactive process between coach and coachee and, in the context of coach development and lifelong learning, between trainer and trainee and supervisor and supervisee.

As has been described in earlier chapters, fundamental to the coaching process is the creation of a learning environment (Carroll and Gilbert, 2011) that enables the coachee to explore presenting issues, goals and contexts from a variety of perspectives in a safe, holding and challenging relationship that encourages the development of self-reflective practice, supports accessing the coachee's own strengths, while also offering the opportunity for broadening perspectives on self, others and systems through the meeting of coach and coachee subjectivities. These principles extend to the domain of coach development and training.

Philosophy of an integrative relational approach to training

An integrative relational approach to coaching as set out in this book seeks to enable clients to make desirable and beneficial changes in their personal and professional lives, develop and grow. It focuses on unlocking and unfolding human potential underpinned by a solid understanding of human experience, adult learning, change theories and system perspectives. It seeks to promote dialogue between psychological understanding and evolving coaching theory and practice, and counter the individualistic tendency in some quarters to split off the discipline of coaching from the wider social and cultural contexts in which human experience and coaching are always situated.

A collaborative-relational orientation to coaching

We have set out that a collaborative, negotiated relationship between coach and coachee stands to significantly impact the flow and outcomes of the work.

Psychotherapy outcome research (Horvath and Symonds, 1991) demonstrates the centrality of the relationship between client and practitioner for facilitating change, as such, training in relational coaching needs to pay attention to the often subtle, yet extremely potent, forces at work in human relationships that influence the ways in which coach and client experience themselves, think, reflect and make meaning together.

Theoretical rigour and critical reflection

In order for coaches to be able to creatively navigate with their clients the challenges of the VUCA world, a sound and critical engagement with theory can provide a solid foundation to practice, enhance coach credibility and confidence in the face of uncertainty and complexity. Western (2013, 2017) encourages coaches to be able to move fluidly between the different coaching discourses (Psy Expert, Managerial, Soul Guide and Network) as different situations require. The same principle extends to all coaching theory, enabling coaches to develop range and flexibility for approaching each unique coaching situation from a range of perspectives.

Theory should not be approached in a dry and abstract fashion, rather, trainees need to be encouraged to pay close attention to how they are making sense of theoretical propositions and, through ongoing reflection and supervision, discover the implications of theoretical ideas for their own practice and vice versa.

From a relational perspective, the most important tool coaches have available to them is themselves. As such, students of coaching need to develop the ability to reflect deeply on their experience, the different ways they are making meaning from these experiences, including different theoretical lenses, and the implications of this for their practice and client situations. Reflection, be it in the moment of working with a client, or in supervision, represents the raw material out of which successful interventions can be designed and executed.

Concern with the person of the coach

Another consequence of the intersubjective emphasis of a relational orientation to coaching is that the person we are is the practitioner we are. Training can provide a theoretical framework along with tools, however, how these are executed, and the impact they have, depends in large part on the person who is the coach. Tutors and supervisors on coaching programmes need to provide supportive and challenging feedback to enable students to know themselves better and become increasingly aware of their resources, their limitations and areas for ongoing development.

To this end it is critical for trainees to experience coaching with relational and psychologically minded practitioners in order to experience first hand the relational dynamics that can unfold for the client as well as the transformative potential of working in this way. It strikes us as a glaring omission that so many coaching programmes do not require coaching trainees to experience being coaching clients outside of structured role-play exercises. This phenomenon can reinforce a subject-object orientation between coach and coachee. By experiencing being a client, coaches are more likely to develop experiential knowledge in service of strengthening empathy and a subject-subject orientation between coach and client central to relational practice.

Supporting the development of unique individual coaching models and identities

An integrative approach supports students to explore and experience a range of theories and practices for coaching and to develop their own coherent approach. Students need to be encouraged to stand consciously in their chosen models, while also cultivating a critical stance towards their orientation as this further supports practice efficacy and impact.

This is a challenging task since it asks of students a commitment to ownership of their own individual coaching model, rather than 'taking on' an existing standard model, and at the same time they need to be aware of developments in coaching research, theory and practice to inform their thinking. This approach, whist challenging, has much to offer on both a personal and a professional level in a field that has thus far (with a few more recent exceptions – see de Haan, 2008; Carroll and Gilbert, 2011; de Haan and Sills, 2012; Western, 2012; 2017) mostly relied on tightly structured models and protocols focused on goals and outcomes, and not on the qualities inherent in the coaching relationship and a sensitivity to the unique intersubjective and contextual dynamics at play in shaping any coaching engagement.

The following guidelines and questions can be useful in enabling coaches to articulate their working assumptions to themselves and facilitate greater conscious ownership of their practice stance.

Guidelines for developing an Integrative-Relational Model of Coaching

Knowing where you stand

- What are the values that underpin your approach to an integrative model of coaching and coaching practice?
- How does your model currently connect with and 'speak' to you personally? What does this reflect of who you are as a person?

Your view of the person/human being

- How do you view the make-up of the person/structure of the person, self and identity? What theories do you draw upon and how do they inform how you experience being with your clients?

- What is your understanding of motivation and what motivates people?
- What concepts inform your understanding of healthy/optimal functioning?
- Effects of context – how do you understand issues of difference-sameness, organisational, social, economic, and political discourses? How do you work with these in your practice?

Concepts that inform your integrative understanding of learning and change

- How do you conceptualise the process of change in coaching? What contributes to the change process?
- How do you think about different personality and learning styles and their impact on coaching and the coaching relationship?
- How do you think about the role of the coach as an agent of change, including aspects of power and hierarchy, and how does this inform your practice?
- How do you think about the different contexts in which coaching happens as well as different types of coaching and their relevance to change?

The process of coaching in the room with the client

- How do you view the co-created coaching relationship? – What is its role?
- What are the features that characterise it? How can it be utilised in service of client development?
- How do you understand the impact of context, multiple stakeholders and work with this?
- How do you currently understand the nature and function of contracting?
- Where do you locate yourself on the intersubjective/emergent – structure/goal continuum? How capable are you of moving along it as different coaching situations may require?
- What interventions, techniques and strategies do you use to facilitate the coaching relationship and the process of change?

These questions, while not exhaustive, serve to invite students and experienced coaches to become conscious of, and reflect on, the assumptions and theories which underpin their practice. They help to develop the ability to account for practice choices, while paying attention to the co-created nature of the coaching relationship, context dynamics and requirements, and developing the flexibility to adjust approaches accordingly. It is important to stress that finding personal answers to these questions is not a 'one off' exercise. In keeping with principles of integration and life-long learning, these are questions that practitioners need to be asking on an ongoing basis and in supervision. This will support practitioners to identify where their practice might have become limited or out of date, and to ensure they are able to learn from those experiences with their coachees that challenge them personally as well as professionally, and which stretch their current working model beyond its current efficacy.

Towards a relational approach to ethics

In this book we have gone to some lengths to describe the implicit impact of individualism, positivism and realism on how coaching as a profession and coaching practices have been construed. Scientific positivism and realism, with their assumption that there is an external reality that can be studied objectively, has been compared with more post-modern perspectives such as social constructionism. Here reality is seen as being constantly constructed and interpreted through multiple discourses and belief systems in ways that are not neutral or objective as scientific positivism would suggest (Western, 2012; 2017; Gergen, 2009; Horkheimer, 1987).

Positivist assumptions about how the world is have given rise to a series of assumptions informing how questions of ethics have been traditionally approached. These have been summarised by Mattingly (2005) as:

(1) It is possible to articulate universal ethical principles or guidelines that are useful in every situation. Ethical rules are context free.
(2) There is always an ethical 'right answer'.
(3) There is an objective position from which to judge what one ought to do. The position is characterised by emotional detachment from the situation.
(4) This objectively defined position, without any emotional involvement, enables the articulation of unambiguous ethical guidelines.

These assumptions are also informed by individualism, the belief in individuals being isolated and self-serving, which calls for codes for guiding the activities and types of relationships of people who as Hinman (2008, cited in Carrol and Shaw, 2013) 'neither know or care about one another' (p. 269). Carrol and Shaw (2013) describe how in the individualist tradition of moral philosophy the concept of relationship is only considered through the lens of social contract theory, which proposes that human beings are independent agents, driven by self-interest, who choose to subject themselves to rules that ensure that all derive some benefits.

Hinman (2008) goes on to describe how the traditions of moral philosophy, which inform many principles and codes of ethics, have not considered relationships, relational contexts nor valued subjectivity. Instead they have tended to privilege reason and have denied any personal connection to the questions of ethics. Feminist philosophers, particularly Carol Gilligan (1982) have argued powerfully that the perspective of social contract theory, with its view of individuals as stripped of emotion and wedded to logic and reason, strips us of those qualities that constitute our very humanity (Carrol and Shaw, 2013). This is further supported by perspectives from evolutionary psychology and neuroscience that demonstrate the central importance of the limbic system in developing and experiencing empathy and connection with others (Azmatullah, 2013; Cozolino, 2006, 2013; Porges, 2011) as well as the critical role of emotions in shaping cognition and thinking processes (Damasio, 2010).

A relational orientation emphasises the fundamental and inevitable inter-connectedness of human beings and, therefore, makes foreground the importance of how people take into account the influences and requirements of relational responsibility, fairness, justice and connectedness (Gilligan, 1992). It raises questions such as how do we balance what we owe ourselves with what we owe others. Carrol and Shaw (2013) stress that without this relational orientation and attention to relational factors 'many important elements are lost, decision making may be flawed or inadequate, and implementation of good decisions may flounder' (p. 104).

They argue that for too long codes and frameworks (informed by the assumptions set out above) have been used as the sole criteria for competency in ethical decision making. While these are important and have their place in developing a degree of ethical competence, these written documents, as argued by Vasquez (2009 cited in Carrol and Shaw, 2013) cannot be a substitute for active, engaged, deliberate and creative approaches to fulfilling ethical responsibility. Rules can be helpful, but are insufficient in dealing with the complexities of everyday life and the VUCA world – 'there will always be too many exceptions to the rules in the shape of particular circumstances and complicating details. Therefore, there is a need for concepts and navigational tools that will assist organisational members in unique situations, which can be understood in different ways and often involve many conflicting considerations' (Haslebo and Haslebo, 2012, p. 28).

Codes and frameworks also perpetuate binary and overly simplified distinctions between good and bad, right and wrong and drive patterns of blame and exclusion. Once we factor in the vital role of context in shaping and influencing behaviour, we see that what might be considered unethical in one context could be justifiable in another. Rules do confer some degree of technical competence, but over-adherence to rules does not cultivate the ethical maturity needed in today's complex environments. Greater ethical reflection is also called for in a relational and post-modern context where individuals (including coaches, coachees and their institutions) are seen as participating in co-creating narratives, realities and behaviours rather than resorting to prior pseudo certainties and assumptions. As Pope and Vasquez (2007) point out, ethical problems often seem to sit in the spaces between the guidelines.

This does not, however, imply moral relativism where any action can be justified. There are still important principles required to guide ethical decision making in complex contexts.

From ethical competence to ethical maturity

It is a feature of transformational learning and adult vertical development (Kegan, 1994; Laloux, 2014) that overreliance on rigid rules gives way to being guided more by principles and embracing a perception of reality that is more complex, where answers to difficult problems and ethical dilemmas need to be discovered on a case by case, situation by situation basis. This takes us beyond the territory of ethical pseudo-competence, based on unquestioning adherence to rigid, presumed to be universally applicable codes, into the territory of ethical maturity involving 'the reflective, rational, emotional and intuitive capacity to decide actions are right and wrong, or good and better; the resilience and courage to implement those decisions; the willingness to be accountable for ethical decisions made (publicly or privately); and the ability to learn from and live with the experience' (Carrol and Shaw, 2013, p. 3).

Writing from within the social-constructionist paradigm, Haslebo and Haslebo (2012) consider a relational approach to ethics as involving abandoning universal definitions of true and false, good and bad, right and wrong, and orienting more to exploring and studying consciously how individuals co-construct meaning, co-ordinate their actions and patterns of relating. They identify what they see as five core concepts that can be used to shed light on these processes. Each has ethical implications for practice.

Context

Is concerned with how in societies and organisations meaning is co-created in unpredictable ways that can never fully be understood by any one individual given the multiple variables at play as we set out in Chapter 5. If we orient to this principle, this gives rise to a 'moral obligation' (Haslebo and Haslebo, 2012, p. 34), which Haslebo and Haslebo see as a social responsibility based on embracing the idea that as humans we are not simply subjected to events but also participate in creating these events. This renders us co-responsible for constructing situations in which all involved can contribute constructively. This has implications for the responsibility coaches and coachees have for co-creating the work and outcomes, as well as raising questions about how each might see the role of coaching and individual change in terms of participating in shaping the organisations and societies in which the coaching is taking place.

Relationship

Drawing on the work of linguistic philosopher John Austin (1962), who demonstrates the relationship building power of language, as well as the work of narrative-based anthropological research, which shows how words take their meaning from their cultural context, Haslebo and Haslebo (2012) identify a particular moral compass point which they call 'the obligation to engage in dialogue' (p. 35). For coaches this implies the need to be alert to the ways in which meaning is being made in the coaching relationship and context, and be willing to explore and question where necessary the efficacy and impact of these processes.

Discourse

This relates to how discourses, the ways in which meaning is made, shaped by culture and history, inform the stories and narratives that operate in organisations and societies. These narratives define and allow for particular positions and possibilities while also limiting others. They determine the roles that individuals are expected to take up such as leader and follower, manager and employee, in-crowd and out-crowd, heroes, villains and victims, to mention but a few of the categories which abound in organisational life. These narratives become like scripts in a play, with set characters and specific scenes, which tightly bound the field of possibility and do not facilitate the creation of new ways of thinking about, and responding to, today's complex challenges. The moral and ethical responsibility here is to pay close attention to how these discourses shape the positions individuals place themselves in (including coach, coachee, context and other individuals) and to assume shared responsibility for ensuring positioning that can contribute to respectful relationships, individual and organisational creativity and flourishing. In Chapter 11 we explored some ways for coaches to engage with questioning dominant discourses where these may be limiting an individual and/or organisations from developing new forms of thinking, relating and acting that might be required to respond effectively to the challenges and complexity of the VUCA world.

Appreciation

Drawing on the work of Dewey (1916) and the philsopher Axel Honneth (1995), Haslebo and Haslebo (2012) highlight the importance of recognition for human beings in order to feel of worth and value. This gives rise to the moral obligation which they term 'inquiry of value to the work community' (p. 224). This involves holding in mind the question of how one's own and others' positions and actions can be of value to the whole work community and society. For coaches this raises questions in relation to the position they take in response to the impact their work and the organisations they work in might be having on societies and the planet, the type of work contexts they choose to engage in and in service of what they choose to engage. It is important that coaches monitor their feelings and choices in relation to the work they undertake and the industries and sectors they work in, as any personal internal conflicts and ambivalence are likely to find their way into the dynamics of the coaching relationship and affect the work and its outcomes.

Power

This is concerned with the fact that different individuals in societies and organisations do not have the same opportunities for having their voices heard and contributing to creating contexts which are creative and constructive. This introduces the moral obligation of helping to create possibilities where leaders and followers, those above in the hierarchy and those below, might come together in mutually respectful relationships, assuming shared responsibility for the cultures, behaviours and strategies they create. This points to a need for coaches to be willing to explore questions of power with their coachees, how they are both enabled and constrained by it, and also find strategies for unlocking, where possible, the collective intelligence of all in an organisation. This is a characteristic feature of post conventional organisations (Laloux, 2014), which recognise that the capacity to lead and follow, depending on individual talent and experience, is not solely related to an individual's position in the organisational hierarchy. This can generate much necessary creativity and flexibility for responding to problems that cannot be resolved through continuing to rely on conventional paradigms and assumptions about roles.

The perspectives we have been setting out in this book point to a world that is far more complex than traditional assumptions about organisations and ethics might suggest. They call for an approach to ethics that moves away from universal principles and guidelines to what Mattingly (2005) terms a 'narrative ethics' whose main objective is to discover what constitutes the 'good' in each unique and specific situation. From a social constructionist perspective, this requires us to explore what stories individuals (including the coach) see themselves as being part of, the network of relationships they consider themselves to be situated within as in Western's (2013, 2017) network discourse, and what future they are trying to build.

Philosophy and practice of a relational approach to supervision

Supervision of coaching is now recognised as being an essential component in ensuring professional efficacy and ethical practice. The supervisory space offers the possibility of a reflective relationship in which to attend to ensuring appropriate boundaries and practices of the profession are respected and adhered to; a space in which the theory and technique can be explored and learnt in order to develop the range and repertoire of supervisees; and a space to reflect on specific client work from a number of angles as set out for example in Hawkin's Seven Eye Model (Hawkins and Smith, 2010), in ways that reveal new strategies and possibilities for furthering the work with clients.

It is particularly important in a relational orientation to coaching to focus on how coaches make more use of themselves as instruments in the process of coaching, rather than an exclusive focus on techniques and strategies. As such, supervisor and supervisee need to co-create a learning environment that provides the space for exploration, discovery and a focus on the 'use of self' in the unfolding relationship of coaching with clients and in their contexts. The supervisory space needs to be one where all aspects of the coaching relationship can be articulated and explored without fear of judgement, to enable supervisees to expand their perspectives and extend their learning. Given the emphasis on use of self and the intersubjective nature of the coaching process as set out in Section 2, this will inevitably include how the coach is being influenced and impacted by the coachee and his context and an exploration of the potential relevance of these resonances for the work. In fact, the principles and practices set out in Section 2 in the context of relational coaching are equally applicable in the context of supervision where, instead of reflection on the coachee's goals and context requirements, the primary task is to facilitate the coach's reflection on client work.

In service of increasing mutuality and conditions supportive of reflection, it is important that supervisors not be seen as the 'experts' who provide strategies for the supervisee. Rather they might be more helpfully seen as the co-facilitators of a dialogue at both implicit and explicit levels of exchange to open up 'new spaces' (Bromberg, 1996) in their and their supervisees' perspectives on themselves, their clients and the contexts in which the work is unfolding.

It can be helpful to think of supervision as a 'play space', in the sense that Winnicott (1971) speaks of the 'potential space between the baby and the mother' (p. 41) in which the child can begin to discover herself in relation to others and the world. He goes on to say '. . . it is play that is the universal, and belongs to health: playing facilitates growth and therefore health; playing leads into group relationships; playing can be a form of communication in psychotherapy' (p. 41). It can also provide a form of communication in relational coaching supervision. As we mentioned earlier, Panksepp's (2012) articulation of the basic motivational systems that all mammals share includes an emphasis on the universality of the play system, 'the joys of rough and tumble play' (p. 22), which he sees as a spontaneous activity done for its own sake and not goal-oriented in the world, at the time in which the playing is occurring. This play system (in a metaphorical rather than a literal sense!) can form part of the supervisory process where we can be encouraged to 'play with' ideas, with possible interventions and ways of seeing options before we make a conscious, adult choice of how to move forward in terms of the current context of a specific coaching situation.

A similar idea is articulated by Ogden (2005) when he describes the supervisory relationship as a form of 'guided dreaming' (p. 1265). Here the supervisee presents the relationship with the client in an evoked, dreamt up, imaginative way. In service of this orientation and fostering of the play space Ogden (2005) states that it is 'important that at least occasionally the supervisor and supervisee feel that they have 'time to waste'. Such a state of mind allows for a less structured, more freely associative type of thinking' (p. 1278). This mirrors in the supervisory context the need in coaching to pause to create space for reflection, associations and 'bricolage' in order for new perspective, meaning and possibilities to emerge.

Ogden (2005) emphasises how the supervisor only hears and experiences second hand the supervisee's experience of the coaching relationship, which forms the material for supervision in the supervisory relational space. Recordings or films of supervision sessions may bring the supervisor closer to a sense of the exchange, but he or she is never in the room with the coach nor in the mind of the coach. It is usually only in training that we have the privilege of being in the room with the coach and coachee during a session and can experience the embodied nature of the exchange, but we need to acknowledge that we are never going to be completely within another's experience even in this context, and the process of supervision will still involve the process of exploration within the play or guided dream space. This attitude supports a more humble, less hierarchical orientation to the supervisee's learning and emphasises the importance of honouring their embodied experience, while encouraging exploration of new ways of being and relating which may have been regarded as too novel or simply irrelevant to them.

Ogden's (2005) position that we may interrupt our dreams in situations that we find difficult, means that supervision can provide a space where the 'supervisee can dream elements of his experience that he has been previously only 'partially able to dream'' (p. 1265). In this sense the 'supervisory session is an informed co-construction created in the medium of words, voice, physical movements (e.g. the supervisee's hand gestures) irony, wit, unconscious communications . . .' p. 1266). This space then allows the supervisee to re-own parts of her experience that she may have been cut off from and gradually open up the relational space for new learning and development.

This means that the supervisor is a co-learner, a co-facilitator of the learning space and not an expert who pronounces on the 'right' strategy. The supervisor, through the lens of being in a supervisory relationship with the coach, attends to the ways in which the coachee 'dreams up' or presents the client, using the same process of embodiment, attunement, resonance and articulation set out in Chapter 8. The supervisor notices what is evoked in him or her and keeps an open mind to the potential relevance of all that is being experienced as simultaneous information about the coach, the coachee, the relationship and the context. The supervisor attunes to the information contained in the ways in which the supervisee embodies and presents the narrative of their client work. In this sense, like the coaching relationship, the supervisory relationship is 'freshly invented' for each unique individual supervisee and client work being brought (Ogden, 2005, p. 1266).

Essential to this transformative learning process is a sense of safety and holding. In essence, 'The supervisory frame is a felt presence that affords the supervisee a sense of security that his efforts at being honest in the presence of the supervisor will be treated humanely, respectfully and confidentially' (Ogden,

2005, p. 1266). Such transformative learning emerges from a creative relational exchange in which the supervisee feels safe. We see this creative process as emergent and opening up new possibilities in complex systems, which we may not have considered before from our present perspectives.

In this process the complexity of the ethical and moral choices facing coaches in complex organisational systems will also form part of the discussion. In this way coaches can be supported to develop the ethical maturity which for Carroll and Shaw (2013) involves a process of development that can be regarded as gradually 'having the reflective, rational, emotional and intuitive capacity to decide actions that are right, wrong or good and better' (p. 137). They add that we need to develop the resilience to implement those decisions and be account-able for these as we integrate these into our 'moral character and future actions' (p. 137). In terms of the ethical complexities of coaching in an organisational context, Carroll and Shaw's (2013) perspective is a resource for the challenging process of taking action, keeping in mind the interests of all stake-holders, as well as our own moral integrity as coaches, in a complex field with varying, at times competing, demands and pressures.

Future frontiers of coaching

Given our interest and experience in the area of coaching leaders in organisations, we have come to consider that executive coaching for leaders can be thought of as a form of supervision as outlined in the relational approach above. Given the complexity that many leaders encounter in the face of an ever-changing global economic and political context, this approach may be attractive as a means for supporting leaders in uncertain times, where they are required to bring more of themselves to work, cultivate and refine their capacity 'to think on their feet' with an ethical orientation. This model is in sharp contrast to a short-term, specific goal-oriented approach to coaching. This proposition has emerged from our experience of coaching senior executives who often require a reflective space, which is not immediately linked to a specific problem or outcome, but more to their leadership role and changing/ever shifting challenges in the wider field in which organisations are situated. It may also serve to challenge leaders in relation to outdated ideas and fears of 'dependency', the lonely hero archetype, and opens up the possibility that leaders and coachees in general might also use coaching as a supportive, challenging 'play space' for increasing responsibility and facilitating reflection in complex dynamic systems. Furthermore, ongoing and regular supervision is a feature of many disciplines where constant change and complexity are the norm, and where there can be personal costs and challenges related to the work. In many ways this describes the reality of many leaders for whom coaching in the form of leadership supervision might provide ongoing support, learning and perspective taking capacity in service of individual, organisational and wider social development.

Organisations providing training in approaches to vertical development and measurement:

Global Leadership Profile: www.williamtorbert.com/global-leadership-profile
Harthill: www.harthill.co.uk
Stages: www.stagesinternational.com

References

Almaas, H. (1996a) *The Point of Existence: Transformations of narcissism in self-realisation*. Boston, MA: Shambhala.

Almaas, H. (1996b) *The Pearl Beyond Price: Integration of personality into being – An object relations approach*. Boston, MA: Shambhala.

Ammaniti, M. and Gallese, V. (2014) *The Birth of Intersubjectivity: Psychodynamics, intersubjectivity and the self*. New York: Norton.

Argyris, C. (1999) *On Organisational Learning* (2nd edn). Chichester, UK: Wiley-Blackwell.

Arieli, Y. and Rotenstreich, N. (eds) (2002) *Totalitarian Democracy and After*. London: Routledge.

Armstrong, D. (2004) 'Emotions in organisations: Disturbance or intelligence', in C. Huffington, D. Armstrong, W. Halton, L. Hoyle and J. Pooley (eds), *Working Below the Surface: The emotional life of contemporary organisations*. London: Karnac.

Armstrong, D. (2005) *Organisation in the Mind: Psychoanalysis, group relations and organisation consultancy*. London: Karnac.

Aron, L. (1996) *A Meeting of Minds: Mutuality in psychoanalysis*. Hillsdale, NJ: Analytic Press.

Aron, L. (1999) 'The patient's experience of the analyst's subjectivity', in S.A. Mitchell and L. Aron (eds), *Relational Psychoanalysis: The emergence of a tradition*. Hillsdale, NJ: Analytic Press.

Aron, L. (2003) 'The paradoxical place of enactments', *Psychoanalytic Dialogues*, 13(5), 623–631.

Austin, J.L. (1962) *How to do Things with Words*. New York: Oxford University Press.

Azmatullah, S. (2013) *The Coach's Mind Manual: Enhancing coaching practice with neuroscience, psychology and mindfulness*. London: Routledge.

Bachkirova, T. (2010) 'The cognitive-developmental approach to coaching', in E. Cox, T. Bachkirova and D. Clutterbuck (eds), *The Complete Handbook of Coaching*. London: Sage.

Bachkirova, T. (2011) *Developmental Coaching – Working with the self*. New York: McGraw Hill Open University Press.

Barber, P. (2006a) *Becoming a Practitioner Researcher – A Gestalt approach to holistic inquiry*. London: Middlesex University Press

Barber, P. (2006b) 'Group as teacher: The Gestalt-informed peer learning community as a transpersonal vehicle for organisational healing', *Gestalt Review*, 10(1), 60–83.

Bateson, G. (2000) *Steps to an Ecology of Mind: Collected essays in anthropology, psychiatry, evolution, and epistemology*. Chicago, IL: University of Chicago Press.

Bateson, G. (2001) *Mind and Nature: A necessary unity (Advances in systems theory, complexity & the human sciences)*. New York: Hampton Press.

Beebe, B. (2000) 'Co-constructing mother-infant distress: the micro-synchrony of maternal impingement and infant avoidance in the face-to-face encounter', *Psychoanalytic Inquiry*, 20(3), 421–440.

Beebe, B. and Lachmann, F.M. (2002) *Infant Research and Adult Treatment: Co-constructing interactions*. Hillsdale, NJ: Analytic Press.

Beisser, A.R. (1970) 'The paradoxical theory of change', in J. Fagan and I. Shepherd (eds), *Gestalt Therapy Now*. Palo Alto, CA: Science and Behaviour.

Beitman, D. and Savenau, R. (2005) 'Integrating pharmacotherapy and psychotherapy', in J. Norcross and M. Goldfried (eds), *The Handbook of Psychotherapy Integration*. Oxford: Oxford University Press.

Benjamin, J. (2004) 'Beyond Doer and Done To – An Intersubjective view of thirdness', *Psychoanalytic Quarterly*, 73(1), 5–46.

Benjamin, J. (2012) 'Beyond Doer and Done To – An intersubjective view of thirdness', in L. Aron and A. Harris (eds), *Relational Psychoanalyis Vol. 4, Expansion of theory*. London: Routledge.

Berne, E. (1966) *Principles of Group Treatment*. Menlo Park, CA: Shea Books.

Berne, E. (1968) *Transactional Analysis in Psychotherapy*. London: Souvenir Press.

Berne, E. (1972) *What Do You Say After You Say Hello?* New York: Grove Press.

Bluckert, P. (2006) *The Psychological Dimensions of Executive Coaching*. New York: McGraw Hill/Open University Press.

Bohm, D. (2002) *Wholeness and the Implicate Order*. London: Routledge Classics.

Boston Change Process Study Group (2008) 'Forms of relational meaning-issues in the relations between the implicit and reflective/verbal domains', *Psychoanalytic Dialogues*, 18, 125–148.

Boston Change Process Study Group (2010) *Change in Psychotherapy – A unifying paradigm*. New York: Norton.

Bowlby, J. (1969) *Attachment and Loss, Vol. 1 – Attachment*. London: Hogarth Press and the Institute of Psychoanalysis.

Bowlby, J. (1973) *Attachment and Loss, Vol. 2 – Separation – Anxiety and anger*. London: Hogarth Press and the Institute of Psychoanalysis.

Boyatzis, R. and Howard, A. (2013) 'When goal setting helps and hinders sustained, desired change', in S. David, D. Clutterbuck and D. Megginson (eds), *Beyond Goals – Effective strategies for coaching and mentoring*. Aldershot, UK: Gower.

Boyatzis, R. and McKee, A. (2005) *Resonant Leadership – Renewing yourself and connecting with others through mindfulness, hope and compassion*. Boston, MA: Harvard Business School.

Bromberg, P. (1996) 'Standing in the spaces – The multiplicity of self and the psycho-analytic relationship', *Journal of Contemporary Psychoanalysis*, 32, 509–535.

Bromberg, P. (2011) *The Shadow of the Tsunami – The growth of the relational mind*. London: Routledge.

Brown, B. (2013) *Daring Greatly*. London: Penguin.

Brown, B. (2015) *Rising Strong*. London: Vermillion.

Brunning, H. (2006) *Executive Coaching – Systems psychodynamic perspective*. London: Karnac.

Buber, M. (1958) *I and thou*. (R.G. Smith, trans.) New York: Charles Scribner.

Buber, M. (1965a) *Between Man and Man*. New York: Macmillan.

Buber, M. (1965b) *The Knowledge of Man – A philosophy of the interhuman*. New York: Harper and Row.

Burr, V. (2003) *Social Constructionism*. London: Routledge.

Carrol, M. and Gilbert, M. (2011) *On Being a Supervisee – Creating learning partnerships*. London: Vukani.

Carrol, M. and Shaw, E. (2013) *Ethical Maturity in the Helping Professions – Making difficult life and work decisions*. Philadelphia, PA: Jessica Kingsley.

Casserley, T. and Megginson, D. (2009) *Learning from Burnout – Developing sustainable leaders and avoiding career derailment*. Amsterdam, Netherlands: Elsevier.

Cavanagh, M. (2006) 'Coaching from a systemic perspective – A complex adaptive conversation', in D.R. Stober and A.M. Grant (eds), *Evidence Based Coaching Handbook*. Chichester, UK: Wiley.

Cavanagh, M. (2013) 'The coaching engagement in the twenty-first century: New paradigms for complex times', in S. David, D. Clutterbuck and D. Megginson (eds), *Beyond Goals – Effective strategies for coaching and mentoring*. Aldershot, UK: Gower.

Cavicchia, S. (2009) 'Towards a relational approach to coaching – Integrating the disavowed aspects', *International Gestalt Journal*, 32(1), 49–80.

Cavicchia, S. (2012) 'Shame in the coaching relationship', in E. De Haan and C. Sills (eds), *Coaching Relationships – The relational coaching fieldbook*. London: Libri.

Cavicchia, S. and Fillery-Travis, A. (2013) 'Coaching at work – A method of facilitating self-directed learning or controlling it?' Middlesex University Research Repository. Available at: http://eprints.mdx.ac.uk/13147/3/Dark%20side%20of%20coaching%20final%20paper.pdf

Chaskalson, M. (2011) *The Mindful Workplace – Developing resilient individuals and resonant organisations with MBSR*. Chichester, UK: Wiley-Blackwell.

Chidiac, M-A. and Denham-Vaughan, S. (2007) 'The process of presence – Energetic availability and fluid responsiveness', *British Gestalt Journal*, 16(1), 9–19.

Chused, J.F. (2003) 'The role of enactments', *Psychoanalytic Dialogues*, 13(5), 677–687.

Clarke, S., Hahn, H. and Hoggett, P. (eds) (2008) *Object Relations and Social Relations – The implications of the relational turn in psychoanalysis*. London: Karnac.

Clarkson, P. (1995) *The Therapeutic Relationship – In psychoanalysis, counselling psychology and psychotherapy*. Philadelphia, PA: Whurr.

Clarkson, P. and Cavicchia, S. (2013) *Gestalt Counselling in Action*. London: Sage.

Clemmens, M. (2007) 'The interactive field – Gestalt therapy as an embodied relational dialogue', in T. Bar-Yoseph (ed.), *Gestalt Therapy – Advances in theory and practice*. London: Routledge.

Clemmens, M. and Bursztyn, A. (2003) 'Culture and body', *British Gestalt Journal*, 12(1), 15–21.

Clutterbuck, D. and David, S. (2013) 'Goals in coaching and mentoring – The current state of play', in S. David, D. Clutterbuck and D. Megginson (eds), *Beyond Goals – Effective strategies for coaching and mentoring*. Farnham, UK: Gower.

Cock, J. (2010) 'Coaching, poetry and inter-relational inquiry', in K. King and J. Higgins (eds), *Organisational Consulting @ the Edges of Possibility*. London: Libri.

Coffey, F. and Cavicchia, S. (2005) 'Gestalt in an information technology organisation – A case study', *British Gestalt Journal*, 14(1), 15–25.

Compernolle, T. (2007) 'Developmental coaching from a systems point of view', in M. Kets de Vries, K. Korotov and E. Florent-Treacy (eds), *Coach and Couch – The psychology of making better leaders*. London: Palgrave Macmillan.

Cook-Greuter, S. (2004) 'Making the case for developmental perspective', *Industrial and Commercial Training*, 36, 275–281.

Cox, E. (2013) *Coaching Understood – A pragmatic inquiry into the coaching process*. London: Sage.

Cox, E., Bachkirova, T. and Clutterbuck, D. (2011) *The Complete Handbook of Coaching*. London: Sage.

Cox, J. (2012) 'Do we understand each other – An inquiry into the coaching relationship when working in different languages', in E. De Haan and C. Sills (eds), *Coaching Relationships – The relational coaching fieldbook*. London: Libri.

Cozolino, L. (2006) *The Neuroscience of Human Relationships – Attachment and the developing social brain*. New York: Norton.

Cozolino, L. (2010) *The Neuroscience of Psychotherapy – Building and re-building the human brain*. New York: Norton.

Cozolino, L. (2013) *The Social Neuroscience of Education – Optimising attachment and learning in the classroom*. New York: Norton.

Crane, R. (2008) *Mindfulness-based Cognitive Therapy*. London: Routledge.

Critchely, B. (2010) 'Relational coaching – Dancing on the edge', in E. de Haan and C. Sills (eds), *Coaching Relationships – The relational coaching fieldbook*. London: Libri.

Crocker, S. (2004) 'Creativity in Gestalt therapy: Book review essay', *British Gestalt Journal*, 13(2), 126–134.

Czander, W. (1993) *The Psychodynamics of Work and Organisations – Theory and application*. New York: Guilford Press.

Damasio, A. (2000) *The Feeling of What Happens – Body, emotion and the making of consciousness*. New York: Vintage.

Damasio, A. (2006) *Descartes' Error*. New York: Vintage.

Damasio, A. (2010) *Self Comes to Mind – Constructing the social brain*. New York: Random House.

David, S., Clutterbuck, D. and Megginson, D. (eds) (2013) *Beyond Goals – Efffective strategies for coaching and mentoring*. Farnham, UK: Gower.

Day, A. (2012) 'Working with unconscious relational process in coaching', in E. de Haan and C. Sills (eds), *Coaching Relationships – The relational coaching fieldbook*. London: Libri.

de Haan, E. (2008) *Relational Coaching – Journeys towards mastering one to one learning*. Chichester, UK: Wiley.

de Haan, E. (2012) 'Back to basics II: How the research on attachment and reflective self function is relevant for coaches and consultants today', *International Coaching Psychology Review*, 7(2), 194–209.

de Haan, E. (2014) 'Back to basics III: On inquiry – The groundwork of coaching and consulting', *International Coaching Psychology Review*, 9(1), 81–91.

de Haan, E. and Sills, C. (eds) (2012) *Coaching Relationships – The relational coaching fieldbook*. London: Libri.

Deleuze, G. and Guattari, F. (2004) *Anti-Oedipus: Capitalism and schizophrenia* (Robert Hurley, Mark Seem and Helen R. Lane, trans.). London and New York: Continuum.

Denham, J. (2006) 'The presence of the trainer', *British Gestalt Journal*, 15(1), 16–22.

Denham-Vaughan, S. (2005) 'Will and grace', *British Gestalt Journal*, 14(1), 5–14.

Dewey, J. (1916) *Democracy and Education*. New York: Free Press.

DeYoung, P. (2015) *Understanding and Treating Chronic Shame – A relational/neuro-biological approach*. London: Routledge.

Dimitrov, V. (1997) Social Fuzziology – *Study of fuzziness of social complexity*. New York: Physica-Verlag Heidelberg.

di Pellegrino, G., Fadiga, L., Fogassi L., Gallese V. and Rizzolatti G. (1992) 'Understanding motor events – A neurophysiological study', *Experimental Brain Research*, 91, 176–180.

Drath, W. and Palus, C. (1994) *Making Common Sense – Leadership as meaning making in a community of practice*. Centre for Creative Leadership.

Eisenstein, C. (2011) *Sacred Economics – Money, gift and society in the age of transition*. Berkeley, CA: Evolver Editions.

Eisenstein, C. (2013) *The More Beautiful World Our Hearts Know is Possible*. Berkeley, CA: North Atlantic Books.

Elkjaer, B. (2005) 'Social learning theory: Learning as participation in social processes', in M. Easterby-Smith and M.A. Lyles (eds), *Handbook of Organisational Learning and Knowledge Management*. Oxford: Blackwell.

Eoyang, G. and Holladay, R. (2013) *Adaptive Action – Leveraging uncertainty in your organisation*. Stanford, CA: Stanford University Press.

Fairbairn, W.R.D. (1953) *An Object-Relations Theory of Personality*. New York: Basic Books.

Farb, N.A.S., Segal, Z.V., Mayberg, H., Bean, J., McKeon, D., Fatima, Z. and Anderson, A.K. (2007) 'Attending to the present: mindfulness meditation reveals distinct neural modes of self-reference', *Social Cognitive and Affective Neuroscience (SCAN)*, 2, 313–322.

Flaherty, J. (2010) *Coaching – Evoking excellence in others*. London: Routledge.

Fletcher, J. (2001) *Disappearing Acts – Gender, power and relational practice*. Cambridge, MA: MIT Press.

Fisher, D., Rooke, D. and Torbert, B. (2003) *Personal and Organisational Transformations Through Action Inquiry* (4th ed.). Boston, MA: Edge Work Press.

Fogel, A. (2009) *Body Sense – The science and practice of embodied self awareness*. New York: W. W. Norton.

Fonagy, P. (1997) 'Attachment and the theory of mind: Overlapping constructs?', *Association for Child Psychology and Psychiatry – Occasional Papers*, 14, 31–40.

Fonagy, P., Gergely, G., Jurist, E. and Target, M. (2002) *Affect Regulation, Mentalisation and the Development of the Self*. New York: Other Press.

Francis, R. (2013) *Report of the Mid Staffordshire NHS Foundation Trust Public Inquiry*. London: The Stationery Office.

Francis, T. (2005) 'Working with the field', *British Gestalt Journal*, 14(1), 26–33.

Frank, R. (2001) *Body of Awareness – A somatic and developmental approach to psychotherapy*. Gestalt Press.

Frankle, V. (2004) *Man's Search for Meaning*. New Jersey: Rider.

Frederickson, B.L. and Losada, M.F. (2005) 'Positive affect and the complex dynamics of human flourishing', *American Psychologist*, 60(7), 678–686.

Freud, S. (1905) *Fragment of and Analysis of a Case Study in Hysteria*. Standard Edition, Vol. 7. London: Hogarth.

Freud, S. (1911) *Formulations on the Two Principles of Mental Functioning*. Standard Edition, Vol. 12. London: Hogarth.

Freud, S. (1923). *The Ego and the Id*. Standard Edition, Vol. 19. London: Hogarth.

Gaffney, S. (2010) *Gestalt at Work – Integrating life, theory and practice*, Vol. 1. Gestalt Institute Press.

Gaffney, S. (2011) *Gestalt at Work – Integrating life, theory and practice*, Vol. 2. Gestalt Institute Press.

Gallese, V. (2001) 'The 'shared manifold' hypothesis – From mirror neurons to empathy', *Journal of Consciousness Studies*, 8, 33–50.

Gallese, V. (2003a) 'The manifold nature of interpersonal relations – The quest for a common mechanism', *Philosophical Transactions of the Royal Society of London Series B, Biological Sciences*, 358, 517–528.

Gallese, V. (2003b) 'The roots of empathy: The shared manifold hypothesis and the neural basis of intersubjectivity', *Psychopathology*, 36, 171–180.

Gallese, V. and Goldman, A. (1998) 'Mirror neurons and the simulation theory of Mindreading', *Trends in Cognitive Sciences*, 2, 493–501.

Gantt, S. and Agazarian, Y. (2005) 'Overview of the theory of living human systems and its systems-centered practice', in S.P. Gantt and Y.M. Agazarian, *SCT in Action – Applying the systems-centered approach in organisations*. London: Karnac.

Garvey, B., Stokes, P. and Megginson, D. (2009) *Coaching and Mentoring – Theory and practice*. London: Sage.

Gendlin, E. (1997) *Experiencing and the Creation of Meaning – A philosophical and psychological approach to the subjective*. Evanston, IL: Northwestern University Press.

Gergen, K.J. (1985) 'The social constructionist movement in modern psychology', *American Psychologist*, 40, 266–275.

Gergen, K.J. (2009) *Relational Being*. Oxford: Oxford University Press.

Gilbert, M. and Orlans, V. (2011) *Integrative Therapy – 100 key points and techniques*. London: Routledge.

Gilbert, P. (2009) *The Compassionate Mind*. London: Constable.

Gilbert, P., McEwab, K., Mitra, R., Franks, L., Richter, A. and Rockliff, H. (2008) 'Feeling safe and content – A specific affect regulation system? Relationship to depression, anxiety, stress and self criticism', *Journal of Positive Psychology*, 3, 182–191.

Gilbreth, F.B. (1911) *Motion Study*. New York: Van Norstrand.

Gilligan, C. (1982) *In a Different Voice – Psychological theory and women's development*. Cambridge, MA: Harvard University Press.

Goleman, D. (1996) *Emotional Intelligence*. London: Bloomsbury.

Goleman, D. (2004) *Emotional Intelligence and Working with Emotional Intelligence*. London: Bloomsbury.

Goleman, D., Boyatzis, R. and McKee, A. (2013) *Primal Leadership – Unleashing the power of emotional intelligence*. Harvard Business Review Press.

Gould, L., Stapley, L. and Stein, M. (2001) *The Systems Psychodynamics of Organisations – Integrating the group relations approach, psychoanalytic and open systems perspectives*. London: Karnac.

Grant, A. (2013) 'New perspectives on goal setting in coaching practice – An integrated model of goal-focused coaching', in S. David, D. Clutterbuck and D. Megginson (eds), *Beyond Goals – Effective strategies for coaching and mentoring*. Aldershot: Gower.

Graves, C.W. (2005) *The Never Ending Quest*. Santa Barbara: ECLET.

Greene, J. and Grant, A. (2006) *Solution-focused Coaching – Managing people in a complex world*. CIPD.

Habermas, J. (1971) *Knowledge and Human Interests*. London: Sage.

Hall, L. (2003) *Mindful Coaching – How mindfulness can transform coaching practice*. London: Kogan Page.

Hamill, P. (2013) *Embodied Leadership – The somatic approach to developing your leadership*. London: Kogan Page.

Haslebo, G. and Haslebo, M.L. (2012) *Practicing Relational Ethics in Organisations*. Chagrin Falls, OH: Taos Institute.

Hawkins, P. and Shohet, R. (2012) (4th Edition) *Supervision in the Helping Professions*. New York: Open University Press.

Hawkins P. and Smith, N. (2010) 'Transformational coaching', in E. Cox, T. Bachkirova and D. Clutterbuck (eds), *The Complete Handbook of Coaching*. London: Sage.

Hay, J. (2007) *Reflective Practice and Supervision for Coaches*. London: Routledge.

Heffernan, M. (2014) *A Bigger Prize – Why competition isn't everything and how we do better*. London: Simon and Schuster.

Hellinger, B. (1998) *Loves's Hidden Symmetry – What makes love work in relationships*. Phoenix, AZ: Zeig, Tucker & Theisen.

Heron, J. (1999) *The Complete Facilitator's Handbook*. London: Kogan Page.

Heron, J. (2001) *Helping the Client*. London: Sage.

Hicks Stiehm, J. (2002) *The US Army War College – Military education in a democracy*. Philadelphia, PN: Temple University Press.

Hinman, L.M. (2008) *Ethics: A pluralistic approach to moral theory* (4th Edition). Boston, MA: Thomson Wadsworth.

Hirschhorn, L. (1998) *Reworking Authority – Leading and following in the post- modern organisation*. Cambridge, MA: MIT Press.

Hirschhorn, L. and Barnett, C. (eds) *The Psychodynamics of Organisations*. Philadelphia, PA: Temple University Press.

Hobart, B. and Sendek, H. (2014) *Gen Y now – Millenials and the evolution of leadership* (2nd ed.). Hoboken, CA: John Wiley and Sons.

Hollis, J. (2001) *Creating a Life*. Toronto: Inner City Books.

Hölzel, B.K., Carmody, J., Vangel, M., Congleton, C., Yerramsetti, S.M., Gard, T. and Lazar, S.W. (2011) 'Mindfulness practice leads to increases in regional brain grey matter density', *Psychiatry Research – Neuroimaging*, 11(1), 36–43.

Honey, P. and Mumford, A. (1992). *Manual of Learning Styles*. Maidenhead, UK: Honey.

Honneth, A. (1995) *The Struggle for Recognition – The moral grammar of social conflicts*. Cambridge, MA: MIT Press.

Horkheimer, E. (1987) *The Eclipse of Reason*. Boston, MA: Beacon Press.

Horvath, A.O. and Symonds, B.D. (1991) 'Relation between working alliance and outcome in psychotherapy: A meta-analysis', *Journal of Counselling Psychology*, 38(2), 139.

Hycner, R. (1993) *Between Person and Person – Towards a dialogical psychotherapy*. Gouldsboro, ME: Gestalt Journal Press.

Hycner, R. and Jacobs, L. (1995) *The Healing Relationship in Gestalt Therapy – A dialogic and self-psychology approach*. Gouldsboro, ME: Gestalt Journal Press.

Isaacs, W. (1999) *Dialogue and the Art of Thinking Together*. New York: Bantam Doubleday Dell.

Izod, K. (2008). 'How does a turn towards relational thinking influence consulting practice in organisations and groups', in S. Clarke, H. Hahn and P. Hoggett (eds), *Object Relations and Social Relations – The implications of the relational turn in psychoanalysis*. London: Karnac.

Jacoby, M. (1994) *The Analytic Encounter – Transference and the human relationship*. Toronto: Inner City Books.

Jenkins, R. (2014) *Social Identity* (4th ed.). London: Routledge.

Johnson, B. (1992) *Polarity Management – Identifying and managing unsolvable problems*. Amherst, MA: HRD Press.

Joyce, P. and Sills, C. (2014) *Skills in Gestalt Counselling and Psychotherapy* (3rd ed.). London: Sage.

Kabat-Zinn, J. (2004) *Wherever You Go, There You Are – Mindfulness meditation for everyday life*. London: Piatkus.

Kaufman, G. (1992) *Shame – The power of caring*. Cambridge, MA: Schenkman.

Kegan, R. (1982) *The Evolving Self – Problem and process in human development*. Cambridge, MA: Harvard University Press.

Kegan, R. (1994) *In Over Our Heads – The mental demands of modern life*. Cambridge, MA: Harvard University Press.

Kegan, R. and Lahey, L. (2009) *Immunity to Change – How to overcome it and unlock the potential in yourself and your organisation*. Boston, MA: Harvard Business Press.

Kepner, J. (1999) *Body Process – A Gestalt approach to working with the body in psychotherapy*. New York: Gestalt Institute of Cleveland Press.

Kepner, J. (2003) 'The embodied field', *British Gestalt Journal*, 12(1), 6–14.

Kets de Vries, M. (1980) *Organisational Paradoxes – Clinical approaches to management*. London: Routledge.

Kets de Vries, M. (2001) *Struggling with the Demon – Perspectives on individual and organisational irrationality*. Psychosocial Press.

Kets de Vries, M. (2006) *The Leader on the Couch – A clinical approach to changing people and organisations*. Chichester, UK: Wiley.

Khrennikov, A. (2014) *Ubiquitous Quantum Structure – From psychology to finance*. New York: Springer.

Klein, M. (1959) 'Our adult world and its roots in infancy', in A.D. Colman and M. H. Geller (eds), *Group Relation Reader 2*. Washington, DC: A.K. Rice Institute.

King, K. (2012) 'The challenge of mutuality', in E. de Haan and C. Sills (eds), *Coaching Relationships – The relational coaching fieldbook*. London: Libri.

Kohut, H. (1977) *The Restoration of the Self*. Madison, CT: International Universities Press.

Kohut, H. (1984) *How Does Analysis Cure?* Chicago, IL: University of Chicago Press.

Krantz, J. (1993) 'The managerial couple – Superior-subordinate relationships as a unit of analysis', in L. Hirschhorn and C. Barnett (eds), *The Psychodynamics of Organisations*. Philadelphia, PA: Temple University Press.

Krishnamurthi, J. and Bohm, D. (1985) *The Ending of Time*. San Francisco, CA: Harper.

Kurtz, R. (1990) (Reprint) *The Hakomi Method*. Mendocino, CA: LifeRhythm.

Kurtz, R. (2008) *Body Centred Psychotherapy – The Hakomi method*. Mendocino, CA: LifeRhythm.

Lacan, J. (2007) *Écrits* (Bruce Fink, trans.). New York: Norton.

Lachmann, F. and Beebe, B. (1996) 'Self and mutual regulation in the patient- analyst interaction', in A. Goldberg (ed.), *Basic Ideas Reconsidered – Progress in self-psychology*, Vol. 12, 123–140. Hillsdale, NJ: Analytic Press.

Laloux, F. (2014) *Reinventing Organisations – A guide to creating organisations inspired by the next stage of human consciousness*. Brussels, Belgium: Nelson Parker.

Lapierre, L. (1993) 'Mourning, potency and power', in L. Hirschhorn and C. Barnett (eds), *The Psychodynamics of Organisations*. Philadelphia, PA: Temple University Press.

Laslo, C. and Zhexembayeva, N. (2011) *Embedded Sustainability – The next big competitive advantage*. London: Greenleaf.

Leary-Joyce, J. (2014) *The Fertile Void – Gestalt coaching at work*. AOEC Press.

Lee, R. and Wheeler, G. (eds) (1996) *The Voice of Shame*. Gestalt Institute of Cleveland Press.

Lee, R.R. and Martin, J.C. (1991) *Psychotherapy after Kohut – A Textbook of self psychology*. Hillsdale, NJ: Analytic Press.

Lehrer, J. (2009) *The Decisive Moment – How the brain makes up its mind*. Edinburgh: Cannongate Books.

Levine, D. (2010) *Object Relations, Work and the Self*. London: Routledge.

Levine, P. (2010) *In an Unspoken Voice – How the body releases trauma and restores goodness*. Berkeley, CA: North Atlantic Books.

Lévi-Strauss, C. (1968) *The Savage Mind (La Pensée Sauvage)*. Chicago, IL: Chicago University Press.

Lewin, R. and Regine, B. (2001) *Weaving Complexity and Business – Engaging the soul at work*. New York: Texere.

Lichtenberg, P. (1990) *Community and Confluence – Undoing the clinch of oppression*. Singapore: GIC Press.

Lines, H. and Scholes-Rhodes, J. (2013) *Touchpoint Leadership – Creating collaborative leadership across teams and organisations*. London: Kogan Page.

Loevinger, J. (1987) *Paradigms of Personality*. New York: W.H. Freeman.

Lorenz, E. (2005) 'Designing chaotic models', *Journal of the Atmospheric Sciences*, 62, 1574–1587.

Losada, M. and Heaphy, E. (2004) 'The role of positivity and connectivity in the performance of business teams', *American Behavioural Scientist*, 47(6), 740–765.

Lutz, A., Brefczynski-Lewis, J., Johnstone, T. and Davidson, R.J. (2008) 'Regulation of the neural circuitry of emotion by compassion meditation: Effects of meditative expertise', *PLos ONE*, 3(3):e1897.

Lutz, A., Greischar, L.L., Rawlings, N.B., Ricard, M. and Davidson, R.J. (2004) 'Long-term mediators self-induce high-amplitude gamma synchrony during mental practice', *Proceedings of the National Academy of Sciences of the United States of America*, 101(46), 16369–16373.

Mackewn, J. (1997) *Developing Gestalt Couselling*. London: Sage.

Mackewn, J. (2014) *Systemic Coaching*. Unpublished Teaching Guide.

Mahler, M., Pine, F. and Berman, A. (2000) *The Psychological Birth of the Human Infant*. New York: Basic Books.

Mann, D. (2010) *Gestalt Therapy – 100 key points*. London: Routledge.

Marris, P. (1996) *The Politics of Uncertainty – Attachment in private and public life*. London: Routledge.

Martin, D.J., Garske, J.P. and Davis, M.K. (2000) 'Relation of the therapeutic alliance with outcome and other variables: A meta-analytic review', *Journal of Consulting and Clinical Psychology*, 68(3), 438–450.

Maslow, A. (1954) *Motivation and Personality*. New York: Harper.

Mattingly, C. (2005) 'Toward a vulnerable ethics of research practice', *Interdisciplinary Journal for Social Study of Health, Illness and Medicine*, 9, 453–471.

McLaughlin, J. (1991) 'Clinical and theoretical aspects of enactment', *Journal of the American Psychoanalytic Association*, 39, 595–614.

McNamee, S. and Gergen, K. (eds), (1999) *Relational Responsibility – Resources for sustainable dialogue*. Thousand Oaks, CA: Sage.

Mead, G.H. and Morris, C.W. (1967) *Mind, Self and Society – From the standpoint of a social behaviourist*. Chicago: University of Chicago Press.

Menzies-Lyth, I. (1960) 'A case study in the functioning of social systems as a defence against anxiety – A report on the study of the nursing service of a general hospital', *Human Relations*, 13(2), 95–121.

Mezirow, J. (1990) *Fostering Critical Reflection in Adulthood – A guide to transformative and emancipatory learning*. San Francisco: Jossey Bass.

Mezirow, J. (1991) *Transformative Dimensions of Adult Learning*. San Francisco: Jossey Bass.

Mindell, A. (2000) *Quantum Mind – The edge between physics and psychology*. Portland, OR: Lao Tse Press.

Mindell, A. (2001) *The Dreammaker's Apprentice*. Charlottesville, VA: Hampton Roads.

Mindell, A. (2002) *Working with the Dreaming Body*. Portland, OR: Lao Tse Press.

Mitchell, S.A. (2000) *Relationality – From attachment to intersubjectivity*. Mahwah, NJ: Analytic Press.

Morgan, G. (1986) *Images of Organisation*. London: Sage.

Myerson, D. (2001) *Tempered Radicals – How people use difference to inspire change at work*. Cambridge, MA: Harvard Business School Press.

Nevis, E.C. (1987) *Organisation Consulting – A Gestalt approach*. Cambridge, MA: Gestalt Institute of Cleveland Press.

Nevis, S., Nevis, E. and Backman, S. (2003) 'Connecting strategic and intimate interactions – The need for balance', *Gestalt Review*, 7(2), 134–146.

Newton, T. and Napper, R. (2010) 'Transactional analysis and coaching', in E. Cox, T. Bachkirova and D. Clutterbuck (eds), *The Complete Handbook of Coaching*. London: Sage.

Norcross, J.C. (2011) *Psychotherapy Relationships that Work: Evidence-based responsiveness*. New York: Oxford University Press.

Nowotny, H. (2016) *The Cunning of Uncertainty*. Cambridge, UK: Polity Press.

Nuttall, J. (2012) 'Relational modalities in the coaching relationship', in E. de Haan and C. Sills (eds), *Coaching Relationships – The relational coaching fieldbook*. London: Libri.

Obholzer, A. and Zagier Roberts, V. (eds) (1994) *The Unconscious at Work – Individual and organisational stress in the human services*. London: Routledge.

O'Connell, B., Palmer, S. and Williams, H. (2012) *Solutions Focused Coaching in Practice*. Hove, UK: Routledge.

O'Fallon, T. (2012) 'Development and consciousness – Growing up is waking up', *Spanda Journal*, 3, 97–103.

Ogden, P. (2009) 'Emotion, mindfulness and movement', in D. Fosha, D.J. Siegel and M.F. Soloman (eds), *The Healing Power of Emotion*. New York: W.W. Norton.

Ogden, P., Minton, K. and Pain, C. (2006) *Trauma and the Body – A sensorimotor approach to psychotherapy*. New York: W. W. Norton.

Ogden, T. (1994) 'The analytic third – Working with intersubjective clinical facts', *International Journal of Psychoanalysis*, 75, 3–19.

Ogden, T. (2005) 'On psychoanalytic supervision', *International Journal of Psychoanalysis*, 86, 1265–1280.

Olalla, J. (2010) *From Knowledge to Wisdom – Essays on the crisis in contemporary learning*. Amazon Media EU Kindle edition.

Oliver, C. (2010) 'Reflexive Coaching – Linking meaning and action in the leadership system', in S. Palmer and A. McDowall (eds), *The Coaching Relationship – Putting people first*. London: Routledge.

O'Neill, M. (2007) *Coaching with Backbone and Heart – A systems approach to engaging leaders with their challenges*. San Francisco, CA: Jossey Bass.

Orange, D., Stolorow, R. and Atwood, G. (1992) *Contexts of Being – The intersubjective foundations of psychological life*. Hillsdale, NJ: Analytic Press.

Orange, D.M. (2008) 'Whose shame is it anyway – Lifeworlds of humiliation and systems of restoration (or "The analyst's shame")', *Journal of Contemporary Psychoanalysis*, 44(1), 83–100.

Oshry, B. (2007) *Seeing Systems – Unlocking the mysteries of organisational life*. San Francisco, CA: Berrett Koehler.

Palmer, S. and Whybrow, A. (2011) *Handbook of Coaching Psychology*. London: Routledge.

Panskepp, J. and Biven, L. (2012) *The Archaeology of Mind – Neuroevolutionary origins of human emotion*. New York: W. W. Norton.

Parlett, M. (1991) 'Reflections on field theory', *British Gestalt Journal*, 1(1), 69–80.

Parlett, M. (1997) 'The unified field in practice', *Gestalt Review* 1(1), 16–33.

Parlett, M. (2000) 'Creative adjustment and the global field', *British Gestalt Journal*, 9(1), 15–27.

Parlett, M. (2015) *Future Sense – Five explorations of a whole intelligence for a world that's waking up*. Beauchamp, UK: Matador.

Pedler, M. (2012) *Action Learning for Managers* (2nd ed.). London: Gower.

Perls, F. (1969) *Gestalt Therapy Verbatim*. Moab, UT: Real People Press.

Perls, F., Hefferline, R. and Goodman, P. (1951) *Gestalt Therapy: Excitement and growth in the human personality*. New York: Bantam Books.

Petrie, N. (2014) *Vertical Development Part 1 – Developing leaders for a complex world*. Center for Creative Leadership White Paper. Available at: www.ccl.org/wp-content/uploads/2015/04/VerticalLeadersPart1.pdf (accessed 14 March 2017).

Petrie, N. (2015) *The How To of Vertical Leadership Development Part 2. Center for Creative Leadership White Paper*. Available at: www.ccl.org/wp- content/uploads/2015/04/verticalLeadersPart2.pdf (accessed 14 March 2017).

Philippson, P. (2001) *Self in Relation*. Highland, NY: Gestalt Journal Press.

Philippson, P. (2008) 'Three boundaries of self-formation', *International Gestalt Journal*, 31(1), 17–37.

Philippson, P. (2012) *Gestalt Therapy – Roots and branches*. London: Karnac.

Phillips, A. (1997) *Terrors and Experts* (reprint edition). Cambridge, MA: Harvard University Press.

Phillips, A. (1998) *The Beast in the Nursery*. London: Faber and Faber.

Picketty, T. (2014) *Capital in the Twenty-first Century*. Cambridge, MA: Harvard University Press.

Pope, K.S. and Vasquez, M.J.T. (2007) *Ethics in Psychotherapy and Counselling – A practical guide* (3rd ed.). San Francisico, CA: Jossey-Bass.

Popovic, N. and Jinks, D. (2013) *Personal Consultancy – A model for integrating counselling and coaching*. London: Routledge.

Porges, S. (2001) 'The polyvagal theory – Phylogenetic substrates of a social nervous system', *International Journal of Psychophysiology*, 42, 123–146.

Porges, S. (2011) *The Polyvagal Theory – Neurophysiological foundations of emotions, attachment, communication and self-regulation*. New York: W. W. Norton.

Rainey Torbert, M. and Hanafin, J. (2006). 'Use of self in OD consulting – What matters is presence', in B. Jones and M. Brazzel (eds), *The NTL Handbook of Organisation Development and Change*. Richfield, NC: Pfeiffer University Press.

Rogers, C. (1974) *On Becoming a Person*. Edinburgh: Constable.

Rowan, J. (2002) *The Therapist's Use of Self*. Open University Press.

Rowan, J. (2010) 'The transpersonal approach to coaching', in E. Cox, T. Bachkirova and D. Clutterbuck (eds), *The Complete Handbook of Coaching*. London: Sage.

Safran, J.D. (1993) 'The therapeutic alliance rupture as a transtheoretical phenomenon – Definitional and conceptual issues', *Journal of Psychotherapy Integration*, 3(1), 33–49.

Safran, J.D., Muran, J.C. and Samstag, L.W. (1994) 'Resolving therapeutic alliance ruptures – A task analytic investigation', in A.O. Horvath and L.S. Greenberg (eds), *The Working Alliance – Theory research and practice*. New York: John Wiley.

Sanchez-Burks, J., Karlesky, M. and Lee, F. (2015) 'Integrating social identities to produce creative solutions', in C. Shalley, M. Hitt and R. Zhow, (eds), *The Oxford Handbook of Creativity Innovation and Entrepreneurship*. Oxford: Oxford University Press.

Samuels, A. (1985) *Jung and the Post-Jungians*. London: Routledge.

Sartre, J-P. (1956) *Being and Nothingness* (H. E. Barnes, trans.). Secaucus, NJ: Philosophical Library.

Sartre, J-P. (1997) *Existentialism and Human Emotions*. Secaucus, NJ: Citadel Press.

Scharmer, O. (2009) *Theory U – Leading from the future as it emerges*. San Francisco, CA: Berrett-Koehler.

Scharmer, O. and Kaufer, K. (2013) *Leading from the Emerging Future – From ego-system to eco-system economies*. San Francisco, CA: Berrett-Koehler.

Schein, E. (1998) *Process Consultation Vol. 1 – Its role in organisation development*. Boston, MA: Addison Wesley.

Schon, D. (1983) *The Reflective Practitioner*. New York: Basic Books.

Schore, A.N. (2003) *Affect Regulation and the Repair of the Self*. New York: W. W. Norton.

Schore, A.N. (2009) 'Right brain affect regulation – An essential mechanism of development, trauma dissociation and psychotherapy', in D. Fosha, D.J. Siegel and M.F. Soloman (eds), *The Healing Power of Emotion*. New York: W. W. Norton.

Schore, J.R. and Schore, A.N. (2008) 'Modern attachment theory: The central role of affect-regulation in development and treatment', *Clinical Social Work Journal*, 36, 9–20.

Schwartz, H. (1990) *Narcissistic Process and Corporate Decay – The theory of the organisation ideal*. New York: New York University Press.

Schwartz, J.M. and Begley, S. (2002) *The Mind and the Brain: Neuroplasticity and the power of mental force*. New York: Harper Collins.

Shaw, P. (2002) *Changing Conversations in Organisations – A complexity approach to change*. London: Routledge.

Shaw, P. and Stacey, R. (2006) *Experiencing Risk, Spontaneity and Improvisation in Organisational Change*. London: Routledge.

Sichera, A. (2003) 'Therapy as an aesthetic issue: Creativity, dreams and art in Gestalt therapy', in M. Spagnuolo-Lobb and N. Amendt-Lyon (eds), *Creative License – The art of Gestalt therapy*. New York: Springer.

Siegel, D. (1999) *The Developing Mind – How relationships and the brain interact to shape who we are*. New York: The Guilford Press.

Siegel, D. (2010) *Mindsight – Transform your brain with the new science of kindness*. London: Oneworld.

Sieler, A. (2010) 'Ontological coaching', in E. Cox, T. Bachkirova and D. Clutterbuck (eds), *The Complete Handbook of Coaching*. London: Sage.

Sills, C. (2012) 'The coaching contract – A mutual commitment', in E. de Haan and C. Sills (eds), *Coaching Relationships – The relational coaching field book*. London: Libri.

Sills, C., Laworth, P. and Desmond, B. (2012) *An Introduction to Gestalt*. London: Sage.

Silsbee, D. (2008) *Presence-based Coaching – Cultivating self-generative leaders through mind, body and heart*. San Francisco, CA: Jossey-Bass.

Skinner, D. (2012) 'Outside forces in the coaching room – How to work with multi-party contracts', in E. de Haan and C. Sills (eds), *Coaching Relationships – The relational coaching field book*. London: Libri.

Spinelli, E. (2005) *The Interpreted World – An Introduction to phenomenological psychology* (2nd ed.). London: Sage.

Spinelli, E. (2007) *Practising Existential Psychotherapy – The relational world*. London: Sage.

Spinelli, E. (2008) 'Coaching and therapy similarities and divergences', *International Coaching Psychology Review*, 3(3), 241–250.

Spinelli, E. (2010) 'Existential coaching', in E. Cox, T. Bachkirova and D. Clutterbuck (eds), *The Complete Handbook of Coaching*. London: Sage.

Stacey, R. (1992) *Managing the Unknowable – Strategic boundaries between order and chaos*. San Francisco, CA: Jossey Bass.

Stacey, R. (2000) *Strategic Management and Organisational Dynamics* (3rd ed.). Harlow, UK: Pearson Education.

Stacey, R. (2001) *Complex Responsive Processes in Organisations*. London: Routledge.

Stacey, R. (2003) *Strategic Management and Organisational Dynamics – The challenge of complexity* (4th ed.). Harlow, UK: Financial Times/Prentice Hall.

Stacey, R., Griffin, D. and Shaw, P. (2000) *Complexity and Management – Fad or radical challenge to systems thinking*. London: Routledge.

Staemmler, F-M. (1997) 'Cultivating uncertainty – An attitude for Gestalt Therapists', *British Gestalt Journal*, 6(1), 40–48.

Stern, D. (1985) 'Affect attunement', in J.D. Call, E. Galenson and R.L. Tyson (eds), *Frontiers of Infant Psychiatry*, Vol. 2. New York: Basic Books.

Stern, D. (1998) *The Interpersonal World of the Infant – A view from psychoanalysis and developmental psychology*. London: Karnac.

Stern, D. (2004) *The Present Moment in Psychotherapy and Everyday Life*. New York: W. W. Norton.

Stolorow, R. and Atwood, G. (1992) *Contexts of Being – The intersubjective foundations of psychological life*. Hillsdale, NJ: Analytic Press.

Streatfield, P. (2001) *The Paradox of Control in Organisations*. London: Routledge.

Strozzi-Heckler, R. (2014) *The Art of Somatic Coaching – Embodying skilful action, wisdom and compassion*. Berkeley, CA: North Atlantic Books.

Taylor, F.W. (1911) *Principles of Scientific Management*. New York: Harper and Row.

Teicher, M.H., Dumont, N.L., Ito, Y., Vaituzis, C., Geidd, J.N. and Andersen, S.L. (2004) 'Childhood neglect is associated with reduced corpus callosum area', *Biological Psychiatry*, 56, 80–175.

Thompson, N. (2016) *The Authentic Leader*. London: Palgrave Macmillan.

Torbert, B. (2004). *Action Inquiry – The secret of timely and transforming leadership*. Oakland, CA: Berrett Koehler.

Tosey, P., Visser, M. and Saunders, M. (2011) 'The origins and conceptualisations of "triple loop" learning – A critical review', *Management Learning*, 43(3), 291–307.

United States Government (2011) 'The Financial Crisis Inquiry Report'. Available at: www.gpo.gov/fdsys/pkg/GPO-FCIC/pdf/GPO-FCIC.pdf (accessed 10 April 2017).

Van Deurzen, E. and Hanaway, M. (eds) (2012) *Existential Perspectives on Coaching*. London: Palgrave Macmillan.

Vansina, L. and Vansina-Cobbaert, M. (2008) *Psychodynamics for Consultants and Managers*. New York: Wiley-Blackwell.

Wainwright, R. (2016) Personal communication.

Wampold, B.E. (2001) *The Great Psychotherapy Debate: Model, methods and findings*. Mahwah, NJ: Lawrence Erlbaum Associates.

Waterfield, R. (2000) *The First Philosophers*. Oxford: Oxford University Press/Oxford World Classics.

Watkins, A. (2014) *Coherence – The secret science of brilliant leadership*. London: Kogan Page.

Watkins, A. and Wilber, K. (2015) *Wicked and Wise – How to solve the world's toughest problems*. Chatham, UK: Urbane.

Watzlawick, P., Weakland, J. and Fisch, R. (2011) *Change – Principles of Problem Formulation and Resolution*. New York: W. W. Norton.

Wellwood, J. (2000) 'Reflection and presence – The dialectic of awakening', in T. Hart, P.L. Nelson and K. Puhakka (eds) (2000), *Transpersonal Knowing – Exploring the horizon of consciousness*. New York: State University of New York Press.

West Churchman, C. (1967) 'Wicked problems', *Management Science*, 14(4), B141–B142.

Western, S. (2012) *Coaching and Mentoring – A critical text*. London: Sage.

Western, S. (2013) *Leadership – A critical text* (2nd ed.). London: Sage.

Western, S. (2017) 'The key discourses of coaching', in T. Bachkirova, G. Spence and D. Drake (eds), *The Sage Handbook of Caching*, Los Angeles, CA, London, New Delhi: Sage.

Wheatley, M. (2001) *Leadership and the New Science – Discovering order in a chaotic world* (2nd ed.). Berrett-Koehler.

Wheeler, G. (2000) *Beyond Individualism – Toward a new understanding of self, relationship and experience*. Cambridge, MA: GIC Press.

Whittington, J. (2012) *Systemic Coaching and Constellations – An introduction to the principles, practices and application*. London: Kogan Page.

Wilber, K. (2000) *Integral Psychology: Consciousness, spirit, psychology, therapy*. Boston, MA: Shambhala.

Willard, B. (2012) *The New Sustainability Advantage*. Philadelphia, PA: New Society.

Winnicott, D. (1958) *Collected Papers – Through paediatrics to psychoanalysis*. London: Karnac.

Winnicott, D. (1965) *The Maturational Process and the Facilitating Environment*. London: Karnac.

Winnicott, D. (1971) *Playing and Reality*. London: Routledge.

Wolf, E. (1988) *Treating the Self.* London and New York: The Guilford Press.

Wollants, G. (2007) *Gestalt Therapy – Therapy of the situation*. London: Sage.

Woodman, M. (1982) *Addiction to Perfection – The still unravished bride*. Toronto: Inner City Books.

Wosket, V. (1999) *The Therapeutic Use of Self – Counselling practice, research and supervision*. London: Routledge.

Yontef, G. (1993) *Awareness, Dialogue and Process – Essays on Gestalt psychotherapy*. Highland, NY: The Gestalt Journal Press.

Yontef, G. (2007) 'The power of the immediate moment in Gestalt therapy', *Journal of Contemporary Psychotherapy*, 37(1), 17–23.

Index

Page numbers in *italics* refer to figures

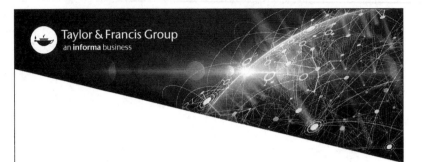